Beyond Diet for Weight Loss

Go beyond just the diet with this revolutionary weight loss program that will shred unwanted weight fast

Introduction

I want to thank you and congratulate you for purchasing the book, *"Beyond Diet for Weight Loss: Go beyond just the diet with this revolutionary weight loss program that will shred unwanted weight fast"*.

Beyond Diet is a type of diet designed to help people lose weight and overcome diseases. It is a specialized gluten free diet that is based on the principles of eating foods with low fat content, foods that maintain glucose levels in the blood, foods with a lower glycemic index and foods that help the body to release insulin. The person who developed this diet is Isabel De Los Rios. She was trained as a nutritionist and later became the co-founder of the Beyond Diet.

The diet is focused on helping people live a healthy lifestyle with fewer diseases and reduced weight. This is an issue that other diets have not addressed. I know you have tried or read about many diets in your effort to overcome weight or prevent diseases. However, Beyond Diet offers you a proven solution to weight loss and disease prevention. By following Beyond Diet, you can easily eliminate foods that are high in calories and replace them with natural and organic foods with fewer calories. However, this whole process takes time and it is necessary to be patient.

Beyond Diet is easy to follow. The diet only introduces a few dietary changes aimed at helping you to lose weight. However, people with some advanced weight gain issues may find it to be ineffective. If you have hundreds of pounds that you need to take off, this diet may not work for you. You may need to stop eating certain types of food completely.

Chapter 1: Why Beyond Diet?

Beyond Diet is considered to be more than a diet. In essence, a diet restricts people's eating habits. Beyond Diet doesn't restrict people, instead it encourages people to eat more. Then why call it a diet? Take an example of a vegetarian. A diet for a vegetarian means consuming foods that do not contain carbs or protein. It includes foods that contain mainly vegetables. You may think that vegetarians are eating only healthy foods but that is not the case. They lack some key nutrients like protein which is essential for the body. Vegans are even more disadvantaged than vegetarians. They cut out all animal products including fish, meat or dairy. Beyond Diet replaces many foods that vegetarians or vegans cut out from their meal plans.

The main difference that you will notice between Beyond Diet and any other diet promoted online is the amount of food consumed. Beyond Diet insists on the importance of eating three meals a day consisting of three classes of food in each meal. It also emphasizes the serving sizes of the meals. For instance, a serving size for a 200 pound person differs from that of a 100 pound girl. Beyond Diet advises people to maintain an appropriate eating pattern, in order for them to feel full and with more energy.

Chapter 2: Beyond Diet Weight Loss Benefits

There is no doubt that the most effective way to help you lose weight is by watching the kinds of foods that you consume. The purpose of this diet is help people abstain from eating processed foods, refined foods and fatty foods that may result in weight gain and cause various diseases. The diet introduces natural and organic foods to help you lose weight and regain vitality.

Beyond Diet helps people to achieve results within the first few weeks. The first step is to determine your body type. You will then be introduced to foods that can help you lose weight. What guides the type of foods to start with is your body type. You are advised not to eat from certain food groups. The purpose is not to restrict you but to give you a customized meal plan to help you achieve your goals.

It is important to remove extra calories from the foods that you eat if you want to fit in a smaller dress size. Why do I say this? Consider the many hours that you spend in the gym to burn the calories that you consume every day. You will find that both exercise and diets are necessary if you want to lose weight. Beyond Diet encourages eating foods with fewer calories in order to prevent weight gain and to promote weight loss. In addition to eating a low-calorie diet, Beyond Diet also encourages eating foods that are rich in fiber and drinking 10 glasses of water. When you follow these guidelines, you will definitely reach your weight loss goal within a short period.

You will realize that Beyond Diet acknowledges, through scientific studies, that each individual has his or her own unique type of metabolism. Metabolism type is the main factor that determines an individual's eating habits and their overall health.

To understand it more, think of this diet in this way. While most weight loss and wellness diets are designed like a groove to fit people perfectly, Beyond Diet is also designed like a groove but can be adjusted to fit any person. You can wear it no matter how uncomfortable you feel but with time you will get used to it.

Chapter 3: Beyond Diet Omega-3 Fatty Acid Benefits

Beyond diet focuses on one nutrient that has numerous health benefits. This nutrient is known as Omega-3 fatty acid. When you follow this diet, you get the following benefits.

1. Pain and inflammation prevention.
Omega-3 fatty acid from fish oil can relieve pain and prevent inflammation. This type of nutrient works through several mechanisms to regulate the inflammation cycle. This cycle is the one that relieves or prevents pain when one is suffering from prostatitis, cystitis or arthritis.

2. Higher intelligence and better brain function.
Nursing mothers or pregnant women are advised to consume foods that contain higher levels of Omega-3 fatty acid. This nutrient help to improve their babies' brain function and intelligence. For adults, Omega-3 fatty acid helps to improve memory, focus, reasoning, concentration as well as learning abilities. Beyond Diet features enough Omega-3 fatty acid for your brain function and intelligence.

3. Prevent depression and uplift mood.
Omega-3 fatty acid from Beyond Diet will not only make you smarter, but can also prevent depression and improve your mood when you feel low. Studies indicate that eating foods that contain enough Omega-3 fatty acid will help to alleviate the symptoms of psychosis, depression, anxiety and bi-polar disorder.

4. Promote cardiovascular health.
Eating food that contains Omega-3 fatty acid has also been shown to promote the health of the cardiovascular system. Beyond Diet features this kind of food. Omega-3 fatty acid helps lower cholesterol, blood pressure, LDLs and triglycerides. This improves your overall well-being and life expectancy.

5. Burn unwanted Body Fat.
Beyond Diet Omega-3 fats can also help to burn unwanted fats in your body. They help regulate the way that the leptin hormone works in the body. This hormone suppresses appetite helping you

to reduce the amount of calories that you consume. It also increases thyroid output which in turn boosts the metabolic processes in the body. These processes enable your body to convert more fats to energy.

You can increase Omega-3 fats intake by eating foods like tuna, salmon, herring, flaxseeds, sardines, pecans, hazelnuts, walnuts, mackerel, butternuts and anchovies. If you find it difficult to get these foods, consider the Beyond Diet. Beyond Diet will increase your daily intake of Omega-3 fats.

Chapter 4: Beyond Diet and Type 2 Diabetes

There are many benefits of a proper diet. Beyond Diet reduces the risk of developing type 2 diabetes. This diet has the potential to help you to shed more than 50 percent of your body weight which reduces the risk of developing type 2 diabetes by almost seventy percent. You will get access to a variety of recipes that reduce type 2 diabetes. These recipes have been created by the Beyond Diet kitchen center and other program members like you. You will also get a free recipe eBook known as 'Desserts Done Right.' This eBook has a collection of 52 dessert recipes that are consistent with your weight loss plan.

Beyond Diet and an Overall Healthy Body

Beyond Diet is focused on helping people have a healthy lifestyle with fewer diseases and reduced weight. The diet offers you a proven solution to weight loss and disease prevention. By following Beyond Diet, you can easily eliminate high calorie foods and replace them with natural and organic foods with fewer calories thus improving your overall health. It is important to remember, however, that this process takes time and it is necessary to be patient.

Beyond Diet can help you to learn about the kinds of food to consume based on your body's metabolic type. This diet can also help you to understand why you are overweight and how you can lose the extra pounds you are carrying. It advocates the use of three aspects of dieting: regular exercise, proper diet and support. Beyond Diet features low-carbohydrate diets, but focuses more on fruits and vegetables, lean proteins and whole grain carbohydrates. This diet does not completely eliminate calories but encourages eating a certain number of calories according to your body metabolic type. Dieters are advised not to eat processed foods. They are advised to eat natural and organic foods.

This diet also comes with a list of recommendations and tips regarding the overall dietary needs and recommended consumption. For example, a simple tip that you can learn from this diet is to drink 10 glasses of water each day when you are trying to lose weight.

Beyond Diet provides you with a free online calorie calculator. This tool helps you determine the types of food that you should consume each day. Using this diet, you don't need to concentrate on counting calories. What you need to do is to watch on the size of the serving in each meal. This tool will help you to understand the percentage of carbohydrates, fats and proteins recommended for your calculated metabolic type.

Chapter 5: Beyond Diet Energy Benefits

Beyond Diet increases energy levels in the body. It achieves this by maintaining the blood sugar levels in the body. People are encouraged to eat three times a day and consume snacks in between breakfast, lunch and dinner. They are also advised to eat immediately when they feel hungry to reduce the risk of overeating and developing cravings for certain foods. You are also encouraged to drink water after every meal. Beyond Diet recommends that people eat foods according to their body size or type. This program employs a step by step guide that starts from finding out the proper body type. To find out your body type, you are asked to answer a set of questions. Once the body type is determined, you are then advised about foods to eat in order to start your weight loss program. If you follow all of these guidelines, you will not feel hungry and dehydrated. You will feel full of energy all day.

Beyond Diet – Benefits of Exercise

Beyond Diet promotes daily exercises as another way to help you lose weight. Exercises are encouraged since they help you to burn fat that may otherwise get deposited in your body. The Beyond Diet provides an easy to follow exercise guides to help you get started on your weight loss journey. There are thousands of weight loss tips that are also offered. These tips help to improve your mood if you feel down. They bring positive changes in your brain. They help fight stress and thus improve your mood. Beyond Diet exercises can also help improve brain functions like concentration, focus, memory, learning abilities and cognition. Aerobic exercises that accompany this diet can help keep the mind sharp.

Chapter 6: Beyond Diet Libido Benefits

Beyond diet can also help to improve your libido and overall body image. Sex and food often go together. So if you want to have fun with your partner, Beyond Diet will definitely help you achieve your goal. There are numerous delicious recipes designed for this purpose. You don't need pharmaceutical drugs to improve your libido. Beyond Diet has a solid reputation and can be a powerful stamina enhancer for your sex needs. Beyond Diet exercise can also help improve your libido. You will find that libido is often affected by self-esteem or mood. These exercises can improve both your mood and self-esteem making you more active in bed.

Chapter 7: Beyond Diet and Sugar Craving

People suffer from sugar craving because of the leptin hormone. This hormone regulates the craving for sweet foods. When sugar is metabolized and stored in the body as fat, it increases the levels of the leptin hormone in your blood. When the amount of the leptin hormone increases over a long period of time, you develop a resistance to it. As a result, your body stops communicating with your brain. You find yourself hungry all the time. Your mouth tells you that all that you want is another taste of sugar or sweet foods.

One factor that contributes to sugar craving is eating foods that are high in fat. Beyond Diet can help you to beat your strong sugar craving and to live a healthy life. This diet features fat free foods and low fat foods. You don't need to pay extra attention to the kind of foods that you eat. Beyond Diet provides you with diet recipes with fewer fats that could otherwise cause a sugar craving. When fats are removed from the foods that you consume, your chances of developing are sugar craving are reduced. Beyond Diet also doesn't contain sweeteners. If you follow a diet that contains sweeteners, you will always need more of it to satisfy you.

Beyond Diet also advocates the incorporation of exercise to beat sugar cravings. When people exercise, endorphin hormones are released into the blood. This hormone gives people a feeling of well-being and satisfaction similar to that experienced when people eat sugary foods to overcome cravings. Beyond Diet exercises can work to overcome sugar cravings.

As you know, maintaining a healthy diet isn't an easy task. It requires people to be careful about what they eat. If you suffer from intense and consistent cravings for certain foods, it is possible you have a deficiency of certain vitamins. Beyond diet can help you to overcome this problem. The diet recommends that people eat three meals a day containing three classes of foods in order to reduce or eliminate food cravings.

Chapter 8: Beyond Diet Gluten Free Benefits

Beyond Diet is gluten free. Gluten is an ingredient commonly found in wheat which scientists say is responsible for binding wheat together. Many people prefer a gluten free diet. This is because some of them are gluten intolerant. This is a condition that causes stomach gas, bloating, intense stomach aches, and diarrhea. For instance, Celiac disease is an adverse gluten tolerance condition. This condition destroys the lining of small intestines making nutrient and gluten absorption impossible.

Therefore, eating a gluten-free diet can be a solution to these conditions. Even if you don't have gluten sensitivity, it is advised that you eat a gluten free diet in order to live a healthy life. You will also realize that gluten is used as an additive when processing some foods. So if you are worried about where to find a gluten free diet, worry no more. Beyond Diet is here for you and can help you to overcome gluten sensitivity.

Beyond Diet Dark Chocolate Benefits

Beyond Diet promotes the eating of dark chocolates. There are several health benefits of eating dark chocolates. The obvious benefit is that dark chocolates are very nutritious. If you consume quality dark chocolate that has significant amount of cocoa, it is very nutritious. It contains several minerals and large quantities of soluble fiber. Studies have also shown that eating dark chocolate can lower your risk of developing heart related diseases.

Diets containing dark chocolate also provide the body with antioxidants. It is manufactured with many organic elements that are biologically active in preventing some of the oxidation processes in the body. These antioxidants include flavanols, catechins and polyphenols. Dark chocolate has also been shown to lower blood pressure and to improve blood and oxygen flow in the body. The cocoa contains bioactive elements that help to improve blood and oxygen flow in arteries that are associated with blood pressure.

Studies have also shown that those people who consume dark chocolate daily have a lower risk of developing cardiovascular disease. The same research also indicates that eating dark chocolate regularly may help protect the LDL that may be otherwise subjected to oxidation. It also raises the HDL, thus protecting it against oxidation.

Beyond Diet Brain enhancement supplements

Beyond Diet Brain enhancement supplements are diets created to boost brain performance, enhance attention and improve memory processes. The diet contains clinically proved ingredients for memory improvement and healthy brain function. The diet contains a combination of powerful ingredients including amino-acids, vitamins and minerals. These ingredients work synergistically to enhance brain performance. Amino acids are used in cells to synthesize protein. They also play a key role in the synthesis process of the dopamine. Dopamine is a neurotransmitter that is linked to an improved learning process, memory and mood. Amino acids in this diet can, therefore, be used against depression, attention deficit, anxiety and mood regulation.

Chapter 9: Is Beyond Diet Right for you?

The straightforward answer for this question is yes. If you have read about dietary programs, a good dietary plan recommends a few basic things as outlined below:

a) It outlines some healthy foods to be included in your meals.
b) It offers alternatives to craving foods.
c) You are able to identify little known "bad" foods.
d) It allows people to develop a meal plan to help them eat well and to stay active.
e) It develops a support system and community to help you achieve your goals.

Beyond Diet has all of the basic things outlined above. It will help you to determine which foods to avoid and help you identify the foods that you should never touch. Beyond Diet does a lot more than that. If you are struggling to lose weight despite the fact that you are exercising and eating right, Beyond Diet is the best diet for you. This diet will help you eat healthy without worrying too much about your weight. If you are also planning to change your eating habits or to incorporate some changes in your meal plan, Beyond Diet is the best approach to help you achieve all these things. If you make a permanent change to the food that you eat, this diet can really be great. People who had adopted the diet and followed it closely not only look better, but also feel better. There are thousands of customer reviews and testimonials posted online regarding Beyond Diet. You will realize that most of these reviews are positive as discussed below.

Advantages of beyond diet

1. Beyond Diet is safe for use by nursing mothers or pregnant women.
2. Beyond Diet allows people to start at their own convenience and to continue at their own pace.
3. It discourages the intake of processed foods, refined foods and sugars but encourages consumption of a variety of natural organic foods

4. Beyond Diet offers a healthy lifestyle and easy to follow approach to weight management.
5. The meal plan advocated by Beyond Diet can be adapted by vegetarians.

Disadvantages

1. Beyond Diet may lead to detox symptoms in some people. These symptoms, though not adverse, range from dizziness, headaches and anxiety to digestive issues especially when you are getting started.
2. Beyond Diet requires that you spend more time planning and preparing your meals.
3. The results take time show up. You may get discouraged if the results are slow.
3. You need to monitor serving sizes closely while on this plan which can be tedious.
4. Low income earners may find organic food expensive.

Chapter 10: Cases Where This Diet Can't Help You

Beyond Diet may not help people with adverse weight and health conditions like obesity. If you're overweight to an extent that you are unable to lift your feet and you want to use this diet to help you lose weight, this diet may not be enough to help you achieve results. You need to consult your doctor because you may be suffering from other health complications. Use Beyond Diet to supplement other weight loses strategies that your doctor might recommend to you.

If you're a heavy drinker or a drug addict, Beyond Diet and most other diet plans cannot work for you. They will definitely pose a challenge. Alcohol doesn't contain many calories but it affects your physiology. With alcohol, no weight loss can occur until you eliminate it completely.

Finally, if you're not ready or realistically committed to adapting the changes that this diet recommends, this diet may not work on you. You may decide to continue with your membership, but you need to stay committed in following and implementing what you learn from this diet. You should take advantage of all the resources available in order to get the best results.

However, if you are willing to make some changes, this diet has a road map for you. The road is easy, flexible, effective and exciting to follow and can surely lead you to reduced weight and a healthy lifestyle.

Conclusion

Beyond Diet is a diet designed to help you lose weight and achieve optimum health over the long-term. Beyond Diet helps people to achieve results within the first few weeks. To start out on this diet, you first step is to determine your body type. You are then introduced to some foods that can help you lose weight. The type of foods to start with depend on your body type. You are advised not to eat certain foods groups not to restrict you but to give you a customized meal plan to help you achieve your goals. There is an excellent research study that supports this diet. You will find supporting videos, an online community, weight tracking guides, food journals, food guides and other features that you won't get from other diet plans. There are also many delicious recipes. They can be used by all of your family members without worrying about gaining weight or developing any future health complications.

The Beyond Diet is not as complicated as other diets that you find on the internet. It is a simple diet that relies on metabolic results to come up with a diet plan. I personally refer to it as a way of life that teaches you the kinds of foods that you need to eat in order to lose weight and stay healthy. There are several key things to be aware of: You choose the right food for your needs that can help you lose weight and stay healthy. The diet is built on principles based on avoiding processed foods, refined foods, sugars and anything that isn't natural. This doesn't mean that the diet only encourages organic foods. Beyond Diet promotes foods that are locally available and that you can afford. This diet is unique in that it doesn't dwell on counting calories but rather using calories to determine the proper food portion for your body's needs. This diet will help you eat healthy without worrying so much about your weight. If you are also planning to change your eating habits or to incorporate some changes in your meal plan, beyond diet is the best approach for you. If you make a permanent change in the food that you eat, this diet can be really great. People who had have adopted this diet and followed it closely, not only look better, but also feel better. If you're looking for the complete, quick and easy to follow package for your weight management, this diets suits you perfectly.

If you enjoyed this book, please feel free to leave an honest review on Amazon.com or by scrolling to the end of this book. Also, check out some of my other popular books listed below in the Amazon Kindle store:

Your Personal 7 Day Raw Food and Drink Detox Guide: Your personal guide to detoxing and using raw foods and drinks.

http://www.amazon.com/gp/product/B00QPOK26W?*Version*=1 &*entries*=0

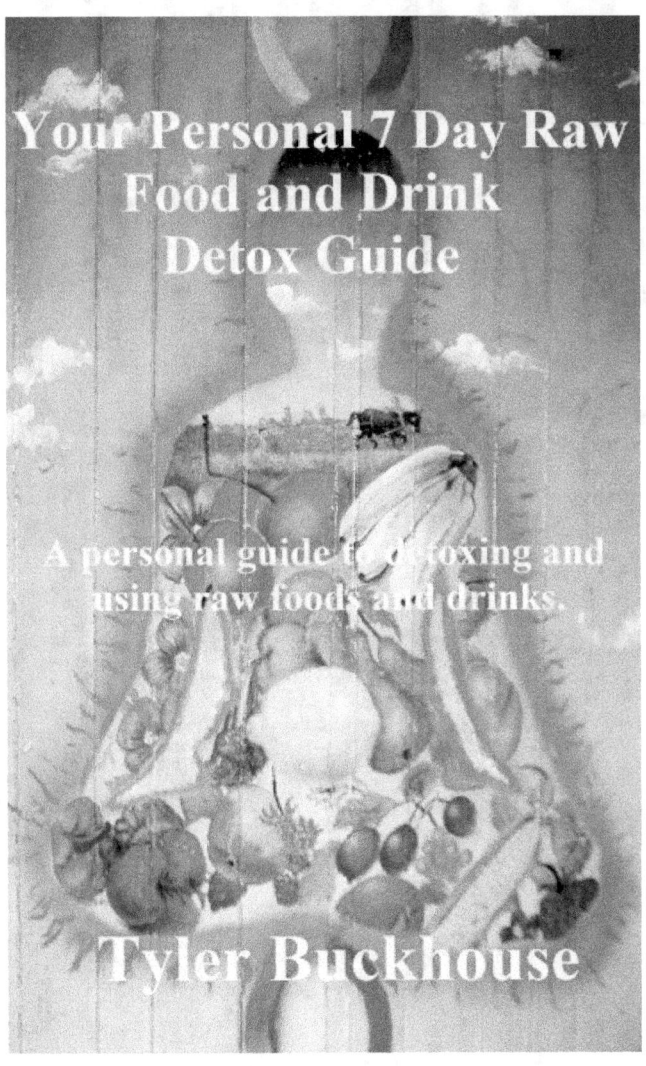

100 Ways to Have Fun at Work: 100 suggestions to help you enjoy work more than you do today.

http://www.amazon.com/gp/product/B00SORU9C0?*Version*=1&*entries*=0

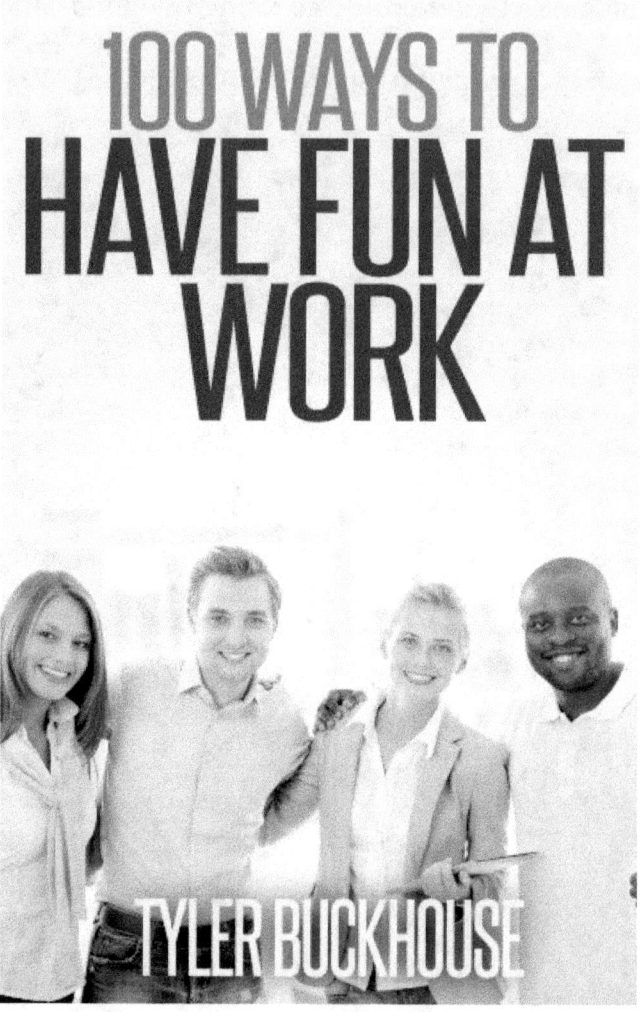

Having Less is More: Minimalist strategies that will improve your focus, time management, relationships, and overall happiness

http://www.amazon.com/gp/product/B0197D6PB8?*Version*=1&*entries*=0

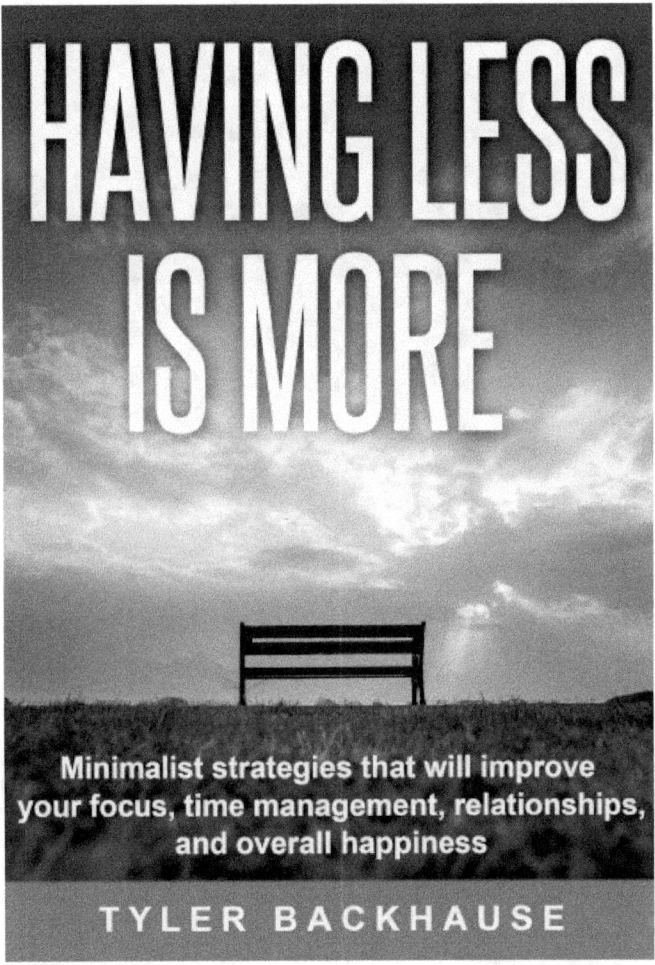

Acknowledgements

A special thanks to my family and friends that have supported me during my transition. Without their help and support, I would have been lost in transition. To my female friends that gave me feminine advice and guidance that has made me the woman I am today. Thank you from the deepest of my heart.

"One is not born, but rather becomes, a woman."

Simone de Beauvoir

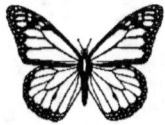

Chapter One

Life as a Boy

I was born in Durban South Africa in 1962, a male named Lee Alexander. I was the last born in a family of five children, to devout Catholic parents. I vividly remember as young as five years old, I became conscious wishing I was born a girl. On one occasion in 1968, my new school friend Mike and I, stood under the avocado tree in our backyard, I looked at him and said: "I wish I were born a girl." I don't know if his reply was to support me or if this were his true feelings, as he replied: "Me too."

Those earlier years, I would look at my three sisters, all older than I am, envious of them knowing that they were girls and I was not. I would read the following nursery rhyme with both utter disgust and envy:

What are little boys made of?
What are little boys made of?
Frogs and snails and puppy-dogs' tails,
That's what little boys are made of.

What are little girls made of?
What are little girls made of?

Sugar and spice and all things nice,
That's what little girls are made of.

It was a simple nursery rhyme; I despised and loved it at the same time. I would read the boy's part only and hate the fact that I was a boy. Why was I made one of these disgusting creatures? Then I would read the girl's only and wish, why was I not made up of sugar and spices and all things nice? I would see pictures of girls in a bathing suit or leotards and ponder at the smooth flatness between their legs and have the feeling that I can only describe as a gut wrenching feeling similar to homesickness. I did not want my male parts in between my legs. I wanted to look the same as these girls. I wanted that flatness with the little slit in the middle.

Growing up I shared a room with my brother, which had an eastern facing window. So for twenty years living in our suburban home, I had the early morning sun. It was a bonus as I would not get heat from the African afternoon sun. My bed was a 3/4 which was in between a double and single size bed, with a wooden headboard and footboard. The walls of our sixteen square meter room were painted navy blue. Like most boys at that time, Bruce Lee was my hero and on my wall, beside my bed, hung the famous poster of Bruce Lee from the movie "Enter the Dragon" with the bloody claw marks on his face, chest, and stomach. He was my inspiration to learn a bit of Kung Fu. I would practice my Kung Fu from a second-hand book I

2

had bought at a local church sale. Kung Fu and Vampire movies were always our first choice when renting movies. In my early teens, we did not have TVs or VHS recorders/player, so you had to rent a 16mm projector along with the large film reels. Some of the movies would require a fine vision lens to play in wide screen.

All my life I had to deal with this transgender issue. A secret I kept locked inside, never to share my true feelings with anyone. Any chance I could get growing up I would sneak into my sisters' room when nobody was home and dress up in their clothes and shoes. It felt so right to be dressed as a girl. I would stare into the mirror as a boy and dislike what I saw. I saw myself as being ugly. I grew up all those years knowing and feeling that I was ugly. Why was I cursed with this body that did not connect to my brain? The internal fight to claim my body was slowly brewing. I possessed a soul that was both male and female. "No, I am a boy" I would tell myself constantly suppressing the female thoughts.

I was fortunate enough never to have been caught cross dressing. But I did come very close once. I was alone in the house, so I snuck into my sister Jean's room that day, my elder sister Alyson was now married and lived just a few blocks away in an apartment. I sat on Jean's bed which was to the left of the door. This way I could not be seen if someone happened to pass by and look in. I slipped on the nylon pantyhose enjoying the silky feeling against my skin. Then slipped on a pair of strappy high heels and secured the strap around my ankles. I looked at them as the sexy sensation filtered down my body.

"Lee, are you here?" the male voice echoed from the back door.

Oh my God! It was my brother-in-law Wayne. I had no time to undo the straps of the shoes and slip off the stockings, so I quickly dove under the bed to hide. I pulled down the pantyhose only to realize I could not take them off as the shoes were secured.

He called out again, as he entered the house and walked down the hallway. I could hear every footstep as he walked down the hallway, the wooden floor creaking with every step. For the life of me, I did not think about locking the back door, though the front door was always locked. I lay still in silence thinking, what I should do? The stockings around my ankles as if my feet were tied together.

"I am here under the bed." I found myself saying.

"What are you doing under the bed?" Chuckled Wayne.

"I am looking for something," I said holding my breath, hoping he would not look under the bed. He just stood in the doorway. "Alyson told me to invite you over for lunch, the food is ready," he said.

"I will be there soon." I nervously replied.

"Ok." I heard him turn around and walk away.

I breathed a sigh of relief. Wow, that was close and I undid the shoes as fast as I could, slipping off the beige stocking. I returned the shoes and stockings in the exact place in the draw, to avoid any suspicion. Minutes later I was sitting at the table with both Alyson and Wayne, realizing how close I came to being discovered. This was my secret I could not afford anyone knowing.

I grew up living a normal boy's life only been attracted to girls. I loved and adored everything about females. I never found myself questioning my sexual preference. In fact, homosexual behavior interests, me but the thought of two women intrigued me immensely. I had my fair share of other boy's or men misreading me, trying to touch me affectionately or suggest I perform a gay act with them. I would immediately turn them down or react in anger. I hated the fact that anyone would presume I was gay. At that time I would wonder why another male would want to be with another male when the female body was so beautiful.

My life as a boy would follow the typical stereotype. We only got TV in the late 70s, so we grew up using our imagination and playing outside. The radio was our only source of audio entertainment, listening to shows like Jet Jungle, Men from the Ministry, Squad Cars and the interesting ghost stories from Ten o'clock tales.

We played games outside like hide-and-seek, cops and robbers, open gates - also known as red rover, haunted house or ghosts, and Cowboy and Indians. We would use broom sticks as horses, and sometimes make a fake horse's tail and place them on the end of a broom stick. Or you could even buy a toy one, which came with a horse's head, and two small wheels at the other end.

One day while playing Cowboys and Indians, a boy named Tony, who was about two years older than me, said, "You are a good cowboy, as you are able to shoot your gun, while riding your horse." His comment did make me proud; but thinking back I recall how difficult it was to hold the broomstick between your legs with one hand, hold a gun in the other hand, and run and shout "Bang! Bang!" and if you felt you had shot the enemy you would say, "Bang! Bang! Bluff you're dead!"

I participated in regular boys sports and played soccer in my younger years. The sporting event I did excel in was the sack race. I would either win the event, or guaranteed to finish in the first three places.

In high school, I played rugby, it was compulsory. I played the position of lock forward. I hated that position as I had to play it because I was a bit taller than most of the boys. Whenever the scrum would collapse, you are the ones right in the middle. I preferred to play flank as that's when the scrum collapsed you could just step aside. I played for the 6th team, which consisted of all the guys that played, not because they wanted to, but because they had to. Our team was captained by Tom, our scrum made up mostly of surfers, stoners, or guys who just did not give a shit about ever winning a game.

Tom would constantly say to us during a game "Come on guys, consolidate."

To be honest, I don't think most of us even knew what the word "consolidate" meant, as we never won a game. Losing games as high as 72-0. Friday nights before the games most of us sixteen or seventeen year olds, would be at the local hotel drinking beers, our 50cc motorbikes parked outside. The next day we would play rugby hungover, listening to Tom shouting out, "Come on guys, consolidate!"

I even took up boxing, mostly for the training. My coach would ask me if I wanted to box in a tournament, but I turned it down every time. I did get pleasure in sparing with the brother of a girl I had sex with. I can't remember why I had it in for him. I just remember getting pleasure from beating him up, until he stopped and pulled off the gloves, refusing to spar with me ever again. One of my school friends, Ed, that I boxed with was even asked if he wanted to be trained to become a professional boxer, but for some reason Ed never pursed professional boxing.

Motocross was another sport I was passionate about. In South Africa when you turned sixteen you able to get a license to ride a 50cc motorcycle. Unlike some of my friends who were more fortunate to have a newer street legal off-road bikes, which we referred to as scramblers. I could only afford a second hand Yamaha delivery bike, the type that had a short seat and a box behind the rider.

I was able to do some conversions to make it look more like a scrambler. I replaced the front metal mudguard with a plastic scrambler type. I had replaced the short seat with a longer one, with a slit cut into my exhaust pipe; this gave my bike a meaner sound to it.

We had our own scrambling track in the bushes not too far from where my friend Grant lived. It was a narrow track with some good turns and bumps. It was not a circular track, but one that had a loop ride back the same track towards the finish. It would end off with a good high jump, in which I enjoyed the brief moment of flying through the air. Because of the design we were not able to race the track at the same time, but instead, we time each other. I was proud to say my timing on my converted road bike was a match for my friend's scramblers. The top bike then was Grant's Yamaha MR50, which would only beat my time by one second. I would dream about actually getting a proper 125cc motocross bike and compete, but it was far too expensive to do.

I must have been about thirteen when I discovered I had semen. I would always wonder what the hype was about "pulling your wire" the term we used for masturbating. Until one day in the toilet, I was excited to see a white cream like substance oozing out the tip of my penis. Since that day like most boys, I would masturbate almost every day. This was not long after I had experienced my first wet dream. That night I dreamt about these sisters that lived two streets away from us. Both very pretty blond girls, Felicity, just had to touch my penis for me to explode into my pajamas pants. That is when I learned what the term "starched sheets" meant.

As the years passed, I would still look into the mirror and not like what I saw. I considered myself ugly. My mother had a saying she would say to me, "You big and ugly enough to look after yourself." I knew it was just a saying, but I did consider myself ugly. This had a profound effect on me, especially dealing with girls. Most of my friends were much better looking than me. I would think that was the reason they would end up having more girls interested in them than me. Looking back on my young life, I would love to travel back in time and find that stupid boy Lee and kick his butt. I missed out on opportunities with beautiful girls. They would show interest in me, but I would pull back thinking I was not good enough for them. How could a beautiful girl be interested in an ugly boy like me? I even missed opportunities to have sex with some of them.

One day I was sitting on the roof of the Bayview soccer club with a friend of mine. His beautiful Afrikaans half-sister Kate was below us. She was about two years older than us and had the reputation of screwing around, mostly with older guys. In other words, she was one horny girl. Her black hair shoulder length, a well-tanned slightly stocky but yet a sexy body.

"Come down Lee, let's go fuck in the toilet," Kate called up to me her brown eyes glistening in sexual desire.

Here was an opportunity I so desired, a chance to have sex with Kate. To this day I could kick myself for not jumping down from the roof and going through with it. Was I just too nervous or was it that I thought she must be bluffing? Who would want to have sex with this ugly boy? The missed opportunity would never be presented again.

Chapter Two

Becoming a Man

I was introduced to sex at a young age. I was only nine when a girl Jane, and I, attempted to have sex. We were the willing guinea pigs, with our peers instructing us what to do as they stood around as spectators. There was no actual penetration, resulting in what is referred to as play sex. I would go onto having one more play sex when I was about fourteen years old. My first real sexual experience would only come when I was seventeen years old with a female in her twenties.

Sex as a young man was enjoyable, for a moment in my life the thought of me wanting to be a girl was a distant thought. Until the day I broke up with my first steady girlfriend, a British hairdresser that was living in Durban at the time. From the start we had agreed that this was not a love relationship, we just enjoyed each other's company and to top it off, the sex was absolutely great. I felt the healthiest in my life at that time and I feel that this helped me do well at technical college. That semester I received four distinctions and was awarded a prize for my results. I was busy with my apprenticeship. Later on in life, I was bound to discover that I would end up having more relationships with hairdressers. I don't know if it was because most of them were more open minded than most other females or that they were more in touch with their femininity that attracted me to them.

The night we broke up, I went straight back to cross-dress, not understanding why I had to feel feminine again. Maybe it was a way I could escape been rejected, feeling the comfort I felt in being a woman. It did not take me long to get back on track. I am fortunate not to let an end of relationship affect me. But the cross-dressing was back in my life. From then on I was able to balance my life both with women in my life and me wanting to be a woman. When with a woman I would keep my secret buried deep inside of me. In some ways being close and intimate with a woman, did bring some relief of my gender issue.

Most of my friends or family would say that I am a lucky person. But I can say that I have had my share of bad luck, but being the positive person I am, I would always try and look at the positive, no matter how bad the situation is. After darkness, there is always light, or after death there is life. There was one episode that happened to me that can either be put down as being just lucky, coincidence or divine intervention.

I was an apprentice at the time and my first car was a light blue mini. Both my front tires were bald, but with my low apprentice pay, I could not afford to buy new tires. I was driving up a hill with some friends on the way to Brighton Beach on a hot summer's day. When "boom!" I had a blowout on one of my front tires. We pulled over to the side to change the tire, right in front of a man sweating as he was mowing his lawn in the hot African sun. He saw our dilemma, wiping the sweat off his brow he walked over to us.

"Do you need some tires for your mini, as I have three Mini wheels. Two of them fairly new and the third partially worn."

Immediately I accepted his offer to buy them for just R40, which was about $20 at the time. This replaced both front wheels completely, and ended up having a good spare. I always thought what was the chance of this happening, talk about a big coincidence. The fact that I had the blowout on that street, and it so happened that he was cutting his lawn at the right time, with the three tires lying wasted in his garage.

I had spent two years in the Air Force, as National Service was mandatory for all white males in South Africa back in the eighties. I earned the rank of Lance-Corporal, possibly because of my unorthodox service to Major Heber.

I was awoken one night by the Major who came into our barracks, shaking my arm saying, "Alexander do you have any pussy books for me?"

I happened to have a novel with me at the time which did have some sex scenes. Amazingly he found a passage that had one sex scene while flipping through the pages after I handed it to him. His eyes lit up with excitement as he read a passage describing a female characters' sexy body.

The Major was an overweight man with a desire to read any book that had sex in it; he probably awarded me the rank because of the books I supplied him to read. From that day on I had preferential treatment and was given the national servicemen's non-profit bar to run. Being the barman for the NS bar made you the most liked, and respected person, on the base. Nobody would dare screw with you, as you had the power to decide to open the bar if or when you pleased. My first call of duty was to raise the price of drinks by a few cents, so that it would pay for my drinks. Six months later I had to give it up; I just could not handle all the heavy drinking and constant hangovers. In the two years' service I had mastered the art of manipulation. If you need something, always offer something in return.

After the two years' service, you were subject to be called up for camps which was either for a month, or you could get called up to serve three months in the operational area, we referred to as the Border. We were indoctrinated that we were fighting communism, not a black/white war. South Africa was at war in what was called, back then, as South West Africa, now known as Namibia. The war took place mostly on the Border between Angola and South West

14

Africa. SWAPO who we were fighting against was backed by Fidel Castro' Cuban soldiers. In 1983 I received my papers to serve for three months.

As a typical boy, I was excited at the chance to go to war, and got the chance to have a license to kill. It was a good feeling being issued the R1 rifle, which was based on the French FN rifle, and having live rounds. The little boy inside you returns, we are playing soldiers for real!

That feeling would change one evening when I was assigned guard duty at the hospital that was located in the Ondangwa Airforce base. The sun had set as I heard the sound of rotator blades from the helicopters. I knew something was going on as I saw the medics and doctors scurrying around. The landed helicopter landed and the doors were opened, stretchers were been wheeled and carried to the hospital with the casavacs; Casavac is a military term used for injured soldiers.

I witnessed both our black and white soldiers bleeding, limbs hanging by threads, open wounds, exposed flesh, and the sound of men dying or crying in pain. This was a wakeup call for me; war was not the fun games you played as boys. This was real; men were severely injured by bullets and landmines. There were so many casualties that some of the men had to be treated out in the open. All surgery rooms were occupied, and at least three amputations took place that night. I could not stomach the sight of all the blood.

The private guard that was on duty with me was curious. He stood on a barrel so that he could look through the window of one of the surgery rooms, to witness a fellow soldier leg being amputated. All the amputations were a result of legs being severely damaged by landmines. I later learned that this battalion was evolved in a heavy firefight referred to as a contact. They had walked into an ambush with landmines in place.

There were trigger happy men among us including myself, due to the curfew at night, you were able to kill anyone that was out after 7 pm. It must have been just after 7 pm one day when I was on duty at the gate. We saw a car driving at top speed towards us. Two of the guys at the bunkers along the perimeter opened fire at the car. One of the guys who shot at the car we called Goofy, as he had buck teeth, who claimed he got buck teeth from a motorbike accident. When the car reached the gate, the man swung open the car door, screaming that he was just a salesman. His leg bleeding from a single bullet wound. Several bullet holes riddled the car. The crazy part was that this was an innocent man; he was just a poor salesman that happened to be on the road after 7 pm. Later on Goofy and the other guy that had fired on the car were arguing about who had shot the man.
"It was my shot that hit him."

"No bullshit it was mine, as I had the right angle."

"Fuck you; I am a better shot than you."

The argument went on for a while, neither one accepting that it was the other who had hit the poor salesman. Only in war can you brag about being the one that injures or takes a human life and have no consequences for your actions.

A few nights later I had a disturbance in front of me as I stood guard in one of the bunkers located all around the base. It was a local residence hut that the noise was coming from. I radioed in the incident and received the reply, "well you know what to do!" Now it was my turn to kill. I cocked the R1 rifle; my thumb hit the switch to rapid fire. The barrel was resting on the sandbag bunker. I looked down the sight, aiming towards the candle-lit hut. Silence surrounded me, only the noise of voices coming from the hut. This was it; this would be my first kill. Was it arguing or just people having fun? There was no time for me to question the noise. There was the curfew, and I had the license to kill. Without hesitation, I squeezed the trigger. There was no loud sound or the kick from the rifle. I quickly cocked it again discharging the first live round. I squeezed the trigger once again. The noise in front of me died down as I realized my rifle had jammed once again.

I often think back to that time, was it divine intervention that had stopped me from possible killing innocent people? Possibly it was a family with children or even a baby. Was it just a family argument under way or just a group of people having fun over a few beers? I do feel at peace knowing that I did not kill that day. Little did that family know that death was at their doorstep that night? Were their lives spared by divine intervention, or was it just the dumb idea that a few of us had, using baby oil to lubricate our rifles? We had a pool on the base we nicknamed Ondangwa Beach. Some of us would use the baby oil to suntan or stupidly to lubricate our rifles. The goal was to go back home with the best tan possible from that desert sun of Namibia. Lesson to any soldier or gun owner: never use baby oil to lubricate your weapon, as it can get sticky.

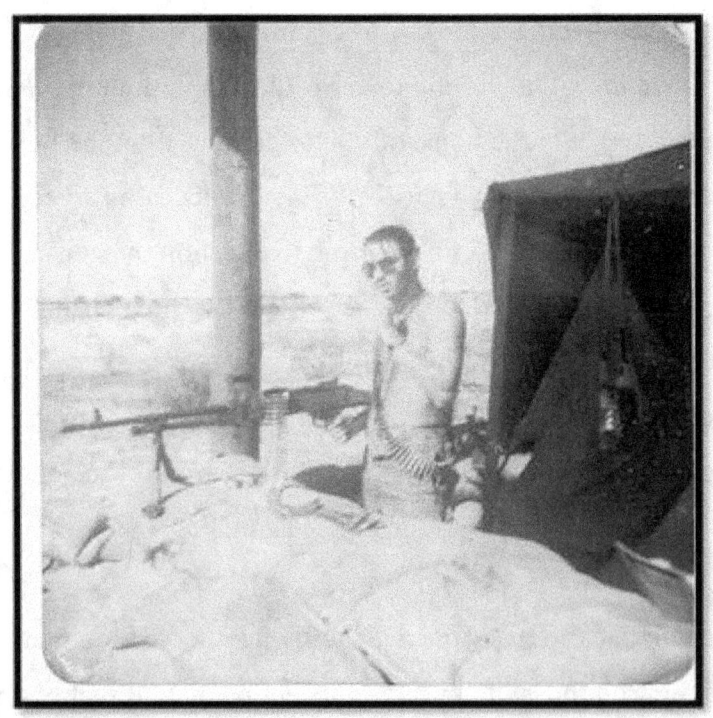

Figure 1, Lee at Ondangwa, Namibia 1983

When I returned home, another bad scenario happened, but I looked at the positive side of it. My girlfriend at the time threw me a welcome home party. Before I had left for the border, I had a farewell party at her house, when our relationship had blossomed. She happened to be my brother in-law's sister Farah. We seduced each other with songs we played on the record player. I chose to play the song by Duran Duran "Hungry like the Wolf". She responded by playing Olivia Newton-John's song "Let's Get Physical." Immediately after the song ended, we headed straight to her bedroom for hours of hot passionate sex. During our time apart while I was on the Border, we fell deeply in love. We wrote to each other every day for the three months apart. But that relationship would end soon after my return.

The night of my welcome home party we had an argument, I don't remember what is was about. Drunk as hell I stormed out into the rain, jumped into my silver Dodge Cold. My foot pressed hard on the accelerator and I headed down the notorious Beach Rd on the Bluff. Reaching the bottom of the hill I hit the pavement on the turn, causing my car to roll a few times. All I could think of in shock while I was rolling was, "Oh my God, I am actually rolling my car." I have heard people rolling cars and dying as the result. Finally, my car came to a standstill. The car landed on its roof, right next to the church, the motor still running. I quickly turned off the ignition in fear the car would catch fire. I crawled out of the window that was shattered, not looking back; I headed to the house in shock. I was fortunate that the only injury I had was a small scratch above my left eye from the broken glass.

A few days later, my relationship ended, and I had received more bad news. My car was not insured. I thought it would have been insured when I traded in my mini for the Dodge Colt. That bad luck turned in a positive, as a few days later I received a cheque from the Air Force for danger pay for the three months I had just served. The amount was just enough to cover the repair cost to my Dodge. Some people would say that was bad luck for losing out on the danger pay. But I look at it as being lucky to have received it to pay for the damage.

In Southern Africa about 1986, when I was working at the Wild Coast, I actually went to go see a psychologist about my transgender identity as I knew it was something that would not go away. The gender identity dysphoria (GID) was part of my life. I just had one session with her. At the time she asked me the question, "How would you like this to turn out?"

I told her I wish it would just go away because that was the easiest solution. But in truth, I knew if I could go to sleep and wake up miraculously turned into a woman. I would have chosen to wake up as a woman.

The lowest point I ever sunk to in my life was when I was working at Sun City. The large casino resort built in a dormant volcano, located in the north-west of South Africa. At that time it was the independent state of Bophuthatswana. I had just left my friend's apartment at night, a couple who were deeply in love. They were so happy and in love with each other. The empty feeling of loneliness overwhelmed me, once again I felt ugly wondering if I would ever find true love like they had.

At this time I had traded in my Dodge Colt for a new white Mitsubishi Tredia SLX. I drove the car up to the top staff parking lot; there was no one in sight. I parked the car, locked the doors and reached for my pistol. I kept in the compartment under the driver's seat. I had purchased the small silver pistol just a year ago for protection, after a horrific ordeal, I went through. The 32 caliber pistol was small, an ideal size that would fit right into my jeans pocket.

This was the first time in my life I had experienced what depression was. I felt so ugly and confused about my gender identity. I decided that day that I would end the mental conflict that was clouding my mind. Cocking the pistol and switching off the safety, I raised my right hand to my temple. "This ends tonight" was my final thought, all I had to do was pull the trigger, and all will be over. At this time the tears were streaming down my face. My quiet sobs soon turned into outright bawling. For minutes I cried continuously, lowering the pistol to my lap. What I did not realize at the time was that crying is actually good for a person. Crying does relieve some of a person's bitterness or sorrow.

With the self-sorrow leaving my body through my tears, a new feeling of self-strength overwhelmed me. I removed the magazine from the pistol and cocked it to eject the bullet that could have ended my life that very night. Since that day I have never steeped that low or ever wanted to kill myself again. Something happened to me that night; it made me a stronger person and even more positive. Maybe it was my guardian angel intervening once again to set me on the right path. Africa was not for me, I needed to find my Island in the sun. An island in the Caribbean would be a stepping stone to me realizing the dream I had as a boy, watching the master view of the slide show of Disney world. My sights were set on one day living in America. I had to leave Africa behind and pursue my dream.

Chapter Three

Island in the sun

The fortune teller Annie that read my cards before I left South Africa
was wrong. She had said that in seven months' time I would find a
very good job surrounded by water, seven months had just passed.
With just three days left before I was to board my failure flight. I
was staying in London, England at the time; my flight back to South
Africa was booked for the upcoming Monday. My dream of finding
my island in the sun or making it to America was not to be.

Then Lady Luck dealt me another good hand.

With just three days left before I was to board my failure flight. I
returned to my temporary home. I was staying with a couple of
friends of mine John and Cindy in a small flat in Ealing Broadway,
London. I climbed up the three flights of stairs to the top floor where
my room was. There on my door was a note left by Cindy. It read:

Lee
Your exciting message is:
Sue phoned & is delighted she managed
to reach you before you fly away.
Please call her urgently
Re. Someone in a casino in South America

is interested in you. She wouldn't

give me any other information.

I said you will call her tomorrow.

tel. xxx xxxx

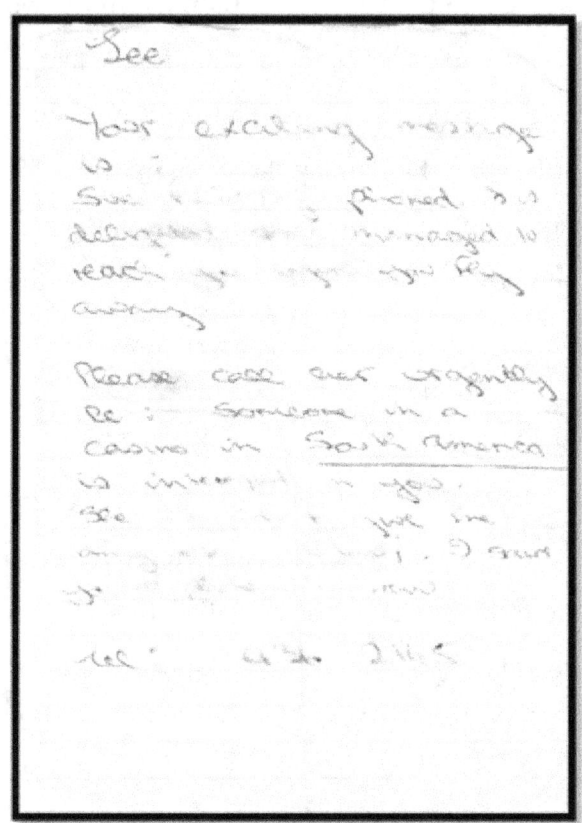

Figure 2 The actual message

In February 1989 I arrived on the Island of Curacao in the
Caribbean. The island would become my home for the next twenty
years. There I met my wife, Sandy. The first time I saw her, I knew

she was the woman I had dreamed about. In the dream, I was wandering through the forest when I came across a beautiful woman by a river washing clothes. Like the 1962 *(my birth year)* song "Patches" by Dickie Lee, I too dreamed of falling in love with a woman from an impoverished country, rescuing her and making her my wife. Little did I know at the time, that our life would resemble this tragedy song in a way I never expected.

My first position carried the title of Chief Mechanic, better known as the Senior Slots Technician. It did not take me long to rise up the ranks in this powerful casino operation. These were my kind of people, well connected. I reached the top of my game answering directly to the five casino owners. The position I earned was: Group Slots Manager. Managing five casino slots operations. I had earned respect on the Island. The locals respectively addressed me as Mr. Lee.

Happy days passed for the next four years until once again I was faced with the scenario of having someone's life in my hands. Like that day in Namibia when I could have killed innocent people. I was given the choice if I wanted the life to end. But this time, it was a very bad person that did not deserve any sympathy.

Sandy and I were in her home country of Dominican Republic at the time. Sandy was about four months pregnant with our son. We received the fatal call at 3 am in the morning. I could read on

Sandy's face it was not good news. Her sweet innocent sister of 16, who had been staying with us in Curacao, had just been brutally raped by the neighbor's son. He had broken into the house, armed with a gun then brutally raped her and forced her to do unpleasant acts that no virgin should ever have done for their first sexual experience. It was so frustrating; I was unable to rush to her side. That morning we rushed to the airport, luckily able to get on the daily flight back to Curacao.

We never went back to stay in the house, instead moved into a Hotel. Where we stayed for three months before I was able to sell the house and move to an apartment. I was approached by a certain person who knew some of the people whose lives were portrayed in the movie "Casino" starring Robert De Niro, Joe Pesci & Sharon Stone.
"Do you want him eliminated? I know someone that can fly into the island, do the job and leave, without any evidence as to who did it."
I could not have someone's death on my conscience, even though I despised the coward that had brutally taken my sister in-law's virginity. The first time is supposed to be a special memory, now she has to live with this ordeal for the rest of her life. The man was convicted and sentenced to jail. While in jail, he was brutally beaten thanks to a certain person I knew, whose lover was in jail at the time.

The first night in the Hotel the three of us sat together on the bed, comforting each other. The three of us had something in common.

Sandy was raped at the young age of fourteen by her stepfather. I mentioned to a female friend later in life that I was shocked to discover, how many woman I had met, that have been sexually assaulted. They were somehow drawn to me, able to confide in me, feeling comfortable to reveal their dark secret to me.

"Oh no, that happens to plenty of women. Many are raped or sexually abused without it being reported, but they live the rest of their lives with the secret in silence" Leah explained.

I too had a secret I was able to block from my memory for all these years. This was also the reason I had purchased a gun for protection back in South Africa. This was the very same gun that could have ended my life in the empty parking lot at Sun City. The traumatic memory came flooding back to me. It was time for me to share them my ordeal.

It happened to three of my friends and I. We were all in our late teens except for Chris who was in his early twenties. Chris, Grant, Ron and I had ventured into the dangerous colored suburb of Wentworth on a Friday night. We went there in search of a shabeen, an illegal place to buy alcohol after hours. We came across four colored men in a car and asked them where we can find a shabeen. They told us that they could get a bottle for us. So we followed them to a house, gave them the money. There was a scuffle at the house by their car, and then they jumped back into the car speeding away, with us on their tail. We followed their car in hot pursuit, driving through the suburb. They finally stopped on top of a hill in a remote area. Chris who was driving parked behind them and exited the car to go ask them for the bottle of cane or for our money back. He soon returned saying that they wanted to have a drink with us. Through the window, I saw one of the men with a machete at his side.

I quickly called to Chris "Let's get the fuck out of here, he has a machete."

The man overheard me and replied, "Don't worry it is just for protection."

Protection from whom? I thought. Chris was a scrawny guy, but when he had drinks inside of him, he had no fear. He said, "Don't worry, we just going to have a drink with them."

Before we knew it, the situation turned nasty, by this time Grant who was sitting in the front seat was outside of the car. One of the assailants swung into to front seat facing Ron and me, poking a knife to my throat. We were forced to give him our wallets. Another assailant who we later learned was the leader of the gang, opened the right back door pulling Ron out of the car. Peter, the gang leader, was a bald, short, stocky light brown skinned man. He forced Ron who was plumpish to the back of the car forcing him to undo and pull down his pant, bending him over. He proceeded to sodomize Ron.

Peter uttered the words I would never forget, "Hey dis oh has shit in his arse."

Why did I trust Chris telling me not to worry? All I could think was this is the night I die, chopped up by a machete.

I looked around we were surrounded by bushes, but I could see a house in the distance. Should I run and save myself, leaving my friends to their deaths?

The man in the front seat came around to my door forcing me out at knife point. As I exited the car, I could see in the corner of my eye Chris on his knees, being forced to give oral on one of the gang members. I was led to the front of the car, should I run was the only thought in my head, death was coming soon with my heart racing. I was forced to do the same. Grant was the only one not molested that night. I often wonder what he was doing while the three of us were sexually assaulted.

Fortunate for us they let us go after the ordeal. We raced to the police station all of us repeating the license plate number of their car over and over so that we would not forget it. The first thing that Chris and I did when we arrived at the Brighton Beach Police Station was to rush to the toilet to clean out our mouths. I washed my mouth out over and over. Two of us were subject to them to them ejaculating their seaman into our mouths. I was so disgusted in what I had to do, constantly spitting all the way to the police station.

We soon learned that the car they were in was stolen. The scuffle we witnessed at the shabeen was the owner of the car trying to escape.

We spent the rest of the night at the police station giving statements. To our amazement, all four men were apprehended while we were giving statements. I remember seeing one of the Afrikaans detectives coming in barefoot in civilian clothes, shirt unbuttoned and the gun just stuck in his short pants pocket. I later learned that a reserve cop that was on duty that night, which helped with the arrests, was Mike. The very same friend I had confessed at the age of five that I had wished I was born a girl. When he recognized that I was one of the victims, he personally made sure that all four men were beating while in custody.

All four were convicted and sentenced to five-year imprisonment. I always wondered how I would react if I ever saw one of those men again. A year later I was given that opportunity as I was walking to work near the train station in Durban. I saw prisoners under tight watch digging ditches along the road. There he was Peter the gang leader, hard at work sweating in the Durban heat picking with hand. Awkwardly all I could do is point at him and laugh at him. He looked expressionless over at me. The four of us never spoke or discussed what had happened to us that horrifying night I don't know if it had any bearing on what had happened to us. But years later Chris and Grant both committed suicide just eight days apart. Both had committed suicide by gassing themselves with their cars.

I was able to shut off this memory, but I think it did have an everlasting effect on me. I don't have any problems with gays. Accepting them for who they are and supporting their way of life. But I detest when a man tries to touch me in any way that can be seen as a gay gesture, even if it is in a way of jest. I know I should not be ashamed of what happened to me that night. There are times when a man has touched me or even put his arm around me when I would react in an aggressive way. I would take offense if anyone referred or associated me as being gay.

Five months later after my sister in-law's ordeal, my son Bret was born. Having a child was the best thing that ever came into my life. His birth even made it to the front page on one of the local newspapers. The hospital had forgotten about me in the waiting room at the time of his birth. I had rented a video camera to record his birth. For hours I was left in the waiting room until my sister-in-law came to find me, hours after the birth. When I finally made it back to the ward, I looked down at my son for the first time. Unconditional love fills my mind and body, it was as if I was looking at a baby me. That moment all the anger at the hospital evaporated away. I was so grateful he was born healthy.

Over the years I would cross-dress whenever I could. Every time Sandy went back to her visit her family in the DR. I would immediately shave off my mustache so that I could transform into a woman for a moment. It surprised me that Sandy never questioned the fact that I had no mustache every time she returned from the DR. I would buy some sexy clothes and shoes, only to throw them away before her return.

I would attend an annual expo in Las Vegas, only to tell my friends and colleague that I was leaving the second day of the three-day expo. The third day was reserved for "Lisa Time"; I would always choose a Hotel that none of my friends were staying at and a hotel that was known to be transgender friendly. When I had the courage, I would wonder around the casino in female form. In a dress with painted toenails, shaved legs, breast forms and a wig I would wonder around playing a few slot machines. I did not get any strange looks, just another tall woman playing the slots. I would also choose a hotel that had beauty salon near the hotel rooms, treating myself to a makeover.

One of my business trips to Puerto Rico I drummed up enough courage to leave the hotel and go to a nearby convenience store. I could not have been too passable at the time. It was the first and only time I have ever heard a man snicker at my looks. Since that day I learned a lot through online research on how to dress to be passable. The key is not to be dressed like a drag queen. Dress for the occasion with the focus to blend in and not to stand out.

After about 10 years, our marriage fell apart which had nothing to do with my transgender identity. It was only after we separated that I told Sandy about my GID. She was quite shocked at first because she didn't suspect anything over the 10 years. She then became very supportive of me. There was a benefit that she did cash in on; the rule was whenever I bought a pair of sexy shoes for myself I had to buy a pair for her. This is one thing I can proudly say about myself, I have an eye for finding sexy shoes. I think that is why we stayed close to each other even though our marriage was over. I felt I had to be there for her too, as she gave me the support I needed.

After a legal separation, I found myself living the single life. Suppressing my GID, I indulged on a sexual rampage having sex with as many women as possible. I was constantly in search for a tall, dark haired woman that would cure me of this gender identity dysphoria. She would be this beautiful feminine woman that would understand me, accepting me the way I am. She would allow me to cross-dress whenever I felt the need to. I would be her male partner and when need be, her girlfriend, to go shopping with or to go out for fun filled nights.

These times took me down a sexual rabbit hole into a wonderland full of sex with Latino sex workers. In my book, I had written as a bucket list item. I self-published the book "Putas of the Caribbean".

Conservatively I had calculated I had sex with over six hundred women. Never finding that special woman I was looking for.

In about 1998, I decided to start laser beard removal in Fort Lauderdale. A decision I would greatly appreciate later on in life. I am so happy I traveled to Fort Lauderdale over the years to do the treatment. I don't know how I managed to handle the pain back then. As the newer lasers, they use now are less painful. It was such a pleasure not to shave anymore. Little did I know back then that my transformation had officially begun. Sandy always told me that if I needed to go pursue my GID further, she would be there for Bret. At that time I still felt responsible to stay and look after my family. Even though we were not the normal married couple, we did stay together as a family.

Chapter Four

Oh Canada

In July 2007, my family and I visited Canada after my application for immigration as a skilled worker was approved. The idea of the visit was both vacation and to enter the country as a Landed Immigrant.

Even though Sandy and I were legally separated, we entered as a family. Our relationship had become one of good friends, almost like a brother-sister relationship. Many of my friends would wonder why we were still together. A nasty comment from a close friend of mine to my ex-girlfriend eventually made it to my ears. "He has no balls to leave her." What I have learned in life, is that everyone has a reason to what others would call their madness. Comments like, "Why are they together? They don't belong to each other."

Why judge people, you never know what their true inner feelings are? Everyone has their own reasons for their own relationships or method to their madness.

We decided to pursue the Niagara area for a few reasons. Sandy had a cousin she had not seen for twenty years that lived there; one of my friends in Curacao was from the area; Niagara Falls had casinos, a possible place for me to work.

Jokingly I said to Sandy and her cousin Liz, "We will only move to Canada if I see a sign. "I have to see a bear in the wild."

Well, destiny was at work once again. We were leaving the cabin we had rented for a few days in Muskoka. Muskoka is a beautiful place up north with scenic lakes and pristine rivers. We were heading back to Niagara; I had given up the chance of seeing a bear in the wild. When all of a sudden I saw through the corner of my left eye what looked like a teddy bear running through the bushes. Immediately I stopped the rental van reversed back to the spot. This was the sign, a whole family of black bears was casually hanging out, some in the trees others roaming around. Canada would become our new home.

I could not resist taking a photo that answered a question a friend of mine back in Durban would constantly use, the saying, "Do bears shit in the wood?"

As opposed to saying, "Yes." I took the photo of the bear shit in the woods and emailed the photo to him with the comment, "Yes they do!"

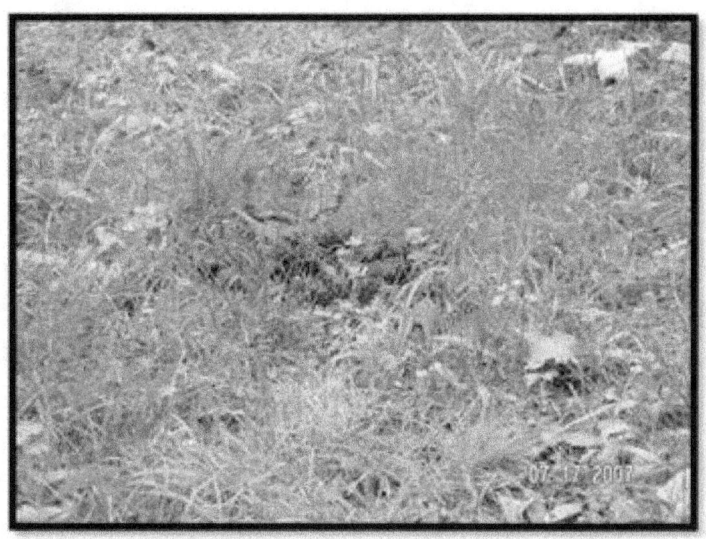

Figure 3 Yes bears do shit in the wood

Later that year we officially moved to Canada. I decided to start my own consulting company, mostly consulting to casinos in the Caribbean. It meant traveling back and forth from Toronto to the Caribbean every month for the next five years. Fun at first with all the travel, but eventually got tiresome.

People in the local bar I frequented would look at me as if I was crazy when I would say, "Shit I have to travel again to the Caribbean." After years of living by the sea, I had reached the point of being beached out.

I sold my house in Curacao, a small bungalow in a resort with a partial sea view. I was the first to buy into the resort, so I was able to make a good profit on the house. With the balance after paying off my mortgage, I bought a townhouse in Canada. A year later we were then able to sell our apartment in the Dominican Republic, with these funds and the help from me, Sandy was able to buy a place of her own.

Valentine's Day 2012 would become a date embedded in my memory for life. Not a day of love, but a day of deep sorrow. I was seeing a woman at the time; we decided to celebrate Valentines on Friday the 12th. That night I passed by Sandy's house to pick up my GPS. She answered the door looking radiant.

"You looking handsome," she said

"You look beautiful." Was my reply

I later found out that she had a female companion at the time. As she closed the door, she turned around to Lucita, "I am happy Lee has found someone, now he won't be alone."

That Sunday on Valentine's Day my son and I went for brunch. That morning we had invited Sandy to join us, but she said she was not feeling well. Sunday was always set aside as our family day, the three of us would normally have lunch together. I thought about buying her Valentine's gift or even sending her flowers but decided not to as I had met someone, and she was also seeing someone. Sending her flowers would have only created confusion or false hopes. Sadly to this day, I wonder how things would have turned out if I had just sent her flowers anonymously.

We arrived at her house with a Burger King take-out for her. There was no reply at the door, even though I had a key to her house; I respected her privacy. After no reply I decided to use my key, calling her name as we entered. Silence filled the house, no TV on or music playing. She loved to listen to her Latin American music. Instinct made me look into the attached garage, her car was there. In the back of my mind, I had the thought that she might try to do what my friend Grant had done, taking his own life by gassing himself in his mother's garage. Her depression was always on my mind as she had tried to take her life twice in the time I had known her. Calling her name once again I went upstairs to the bedrooms, she was not there. As I returned to the main level, Bret decided to down into the basement to look at the salon she and I had recently set up. It was that coming week that she would open her hair salon offering, hairdressing, and waxing.

"FUCK!" I heard Bret screaming from the basement and then heard the thud as he punched the wall. Quickly I ran down the stairs as he passed by me rushing upstairs. Immediately I knew I was about to see something I had dreaded all these years, but somehow known that this day could come.

As I stepped down from the second flight of stairs, I can only explain it like walking into a horror movie. My immediate shocking thought was, "You actually did it!"

She would often tell me her sad dream of wanting to depart from this world. No matter how I tried to tell her that there are people in this world with worse lives than what she had, Sandy so wanted to join her mother she had lost to cancer just after we married.

That image will forever be etched into my brain. Her lifeless body hung at the end of a scarf. Her right leg bent backward, the left forward, almost as if she was in a sitting position. She was dressed in a simple floral short dress; her legs showed no color as if no blood was flowing through her lifeless body. It was only after all the investigation that ruled out foul play, that the detective explained to me how or why her legs were touching the floor. It was the weight of her body that had stretched the scarf, lowering her body to the position I had found her.

I rushed to her the thought racing through my mind, "What do I do? Do I leave her like this for the police to see?"
My survival instincts immediately kicked in. Super strength embodied me, with my left hand I grabbed onto the scarf lifting her body. Somehow I was able to hold the weight of her body with my left hand as my right had miraculously untied the scarf from the beam. I lay her on her back loosening the scarf around her neck.
I reached for the cordless phone in the basement frantically calling 911. For a brief moment, I could not reach them, or I was doing something wrong in trying to make the call. So I attempted to give

her CPR I had learned in my teenage years. This was the first time in my life I had to give it. My lungs full of air I blew into her mouth. Her chest rose up as her lungs filled with some air, but the air was escaping from her nose. Then I proceeded to give her short heart pumps. I tried calling 911 again, this time, I got through, I can't remember the exact words I frantically said to the 911 operator, it went something like this.

"My wife tried to commit suicide by hanging herself, she's not breathing!"

Calmly and professionally the operator instructed me to the correct way of CPR. About 15 heart pumps to a few mouth to mouth breathing. Making sure to block her nose. I placed the phone down, my head spinning with the adrenalin pumping. "How many heart pumps?"

I had to pick up the phone again. Sandy's life was in my hands. "Please breathe." The thoughts were screaming in my mind, going through the routine of heart pumps and mouth to mouth resuscitation.

I was disrupted by the doorbell ringing, what turned out to be just five minutes after I placed the 911 call. I called up to Bret to let them into the house. As soon as I saw the blue uniformed man come down, I stopped the CPR, picked up the phone and said to the operator, "They are here." and then closed the phone stepping back. But I realized it was a policeman. Who immediately helped by doing

41

the heart pumps while I applied the mouth to mouth. I exhaled all the air I could into Sandy's lungs lifting up to gasp for air. But instead of breathing in fresh air I breathed in the same air expelled from her lungs. Nausea kicked in, I moved back on my knees trying my utmost not to throw up.

"Pull yourself together," My subconscious mind was telling me. "You have to save her life." I got a hold of myself forcing myself to concentrate on the urgent task at hand. Force-swallowing the vomit back I was able to continue the mouth to mouth.

There was still no sign of life as the paramedics soon arrived. I retreated upstairs to join Bret who sat on the couch. The only thing he could say to me was, "I will never forget what I just saw."

I tried my best to console him, there were no tears being shed by either of us, both still in shock. The policeman came to us numerous times asking what had happened. Only to realize after the fact that, this is part of their policy to make sure there are no discrepancies, after all, I am the separated husband.

The policeman would come up once again from the basement and said to me, "We have her breathing on her own; your CPR might have saved her life."

For a moment all my worries disappeared. I hugged my son and said, "She is going to be okay." On the way to the hospital, the thought of brain damage seeped in. "You know that she could have brain damage," I explained to Bret.

When we reached the hospital, they let me park by the emergency entrance. We were then led to a small waiting room. I have to say that, in Canada, the emergency personnel all handled this in a professional and caring way. Support workers were there in the waiting room offering me their support.

The temporary hope was soon dashed when the doctor entered the room. He was cordial but direct and to the point. "The situation is not good; your wife had two cardiac arrests on the way to the hospital."

Only then did it hit me I was losing the woman I still loved, the mother of my child, my best friend. I broke down crying holding tight onto my son's hand. Trying to hold back the tears I said to the Doctor, "I have to see Sandy."

At this time she was still on the main level of the St Catharines General Hospital. My son did not want to go into the ward. There lay Sandy her eyes covered with patches, her chest rising up and down to the rhythm of the machine that breathed life into her.

Holding her warm hand I pleaded with her, "Please fight for your son, please wake up."

What I realized now, thinking back, I should have said to her, "Sandy, please fight for me, wake for me, I don't want you to die." On the John Tesh radio show, he had mentioned this is how you can save a person from committing suicide, by telling them you don't want them to die.

Sandy was moved upstairs to the ICU ward, by this time her cousin and friends had arrived. The moment was so surreal as I walked along the clean well-corridor. I thought, "This is not a movie, TV show, or some soap opera happening. This is real!"

Sandy loved her soap operas known in Spanish as "*Telenovelas*," the Latin American people lived passionate and emotional lives.

The same policeman that was first on the scene was there the entire time. Another Doctor soon came in to deliver more bad news, as a result of a brain scan. "She is stable, but there is only one vital signal from her brain, where there should be five."

There were people from the organ donation society asking me if I would consent to her organs been donated? I knew that Sandy would have liked this, knowing that in death she was able to save another life.

Even after this news, I was still holding out hope, once again I broke down crying. At this time the policeman and support workers left the waiting room to give us time to ourselves. It was decided that I could go home as they have to wait twenty-four hours to see if there is any change in her condition. Before the support workers left, they handed me a package of documentation.

I arrived home and found myself opening my closet door. It was time for me to talk to God. I stood motionless staring blankly into the closet. "Dear God if it means we have to make our marriage work to save Sandy's life. I choose my family over everything, give me back my Sandy, and I will make the marriage work."

Sadly I knew, in the back of my mind, it was over. Sandy would not fight to survive, why would she return to a world she thought was too difficult for her. She was finally off to reunite with her loving mother she had missed all these years.

In the early hours of the morning I received a call from the hospital. Sandy's situation had turned for the worst. By Eight O'clock, I had to return to the hospital as the twenty- fourth hour was approaching. This time, I was alone in the waiting room with an older woman whose sister was in ICU with complications with her liver. We chatted for a while both comforted each other, hoping for the best outcome for both of us. As a catholic, you were taught that any person that commits suicide would go to hell. She comforted me by saying, "Maybe at the time of her hanging herself, your wife regretted doing it." I don't believe in Catholic teachings on this point. Depression is a sickness, the chemical imbalance in your body can make you do things you would not do with a sound mind.

A young male nurse came to speak to me about Sandy. He was asking me if I wanted them to revive Sandy if she goes into another cardiac arrest. I felt like screaming to this nurse to, "Shut the fuck up!" As he talked and talked. How can he force to play God on life?

Sandy's family would resent me for making this decision even though I knew Sandy would have preferred me to take her off life support. We were still legally married according to Canada, so I had become her legal guardian. I was the only one authorized to make these difficult decisions.

Later that morning her cousin and friends arrived at about 10am, we delivered the news that her body was shutting down. A Catholic priest was on site to perform her last rights. It all came down to me making the final decision of whether to have her taken off life support or not. I looked around the room to her friends and only other family member present; her cousin Liz. I could see in all their teary eyes it was time for me to make the decision. Even the priest gave me his support. It was time to release her to the afterlife.
We all went into the ward to say our final farewell. Liz was screaming in Spanish, "Wake up Sandy, for God's sake wake up!"
I held Sandy's hand for the last time, it was now cold, no sign of life. Leaning over I kissed her goodbye promising her that I would look after our son and that we will meet again someday in paradise."
The priest said a final prayer then we all left the room. In the privacy of just the medical staff Sandy's life support was shut down. We were allowed back into the room one more time. I looked down at Sandy, tears flowing from my eyes. She lay peacefully motionless, the machine that kept her breathing now stood silently by her side.

My dear wife, friend, partner and mother of my only child would now just be present in my memories.

I arrived home and met my son in the hallway, hugging him I said, "It's over, she's gone." We hugged each other for a moment, father and son alone in this world. I went upstairs to my room, opened the package the support workers had left me. It contained books and documents offering support in a time of grief.

The weeks and months that followed Sandy's death were the toughest I ever had to endure. I felt so much guilt for her death. There were thousands of ways I could have saved her life, had we got there just a few minutes early; said the right things or told her what I wanted to tell her just a few weeks before her death. "Sandy if there was the choice of being single and free or making our marriage work again. I would prefer the latter. Family is more important than anything I can imagine."

So my advice to anyone that feels they need to say something to a loved one. Do it now as you will never know when a moment in time will be the last time you see each other. At least my last memory of us together was a pleasant one her final words to me, "You look handsome tonight" and my final words to her "You look beautiful."

My life had become like a spinning compass with no direction. I had to learn quickly to become both mother and father to my son. I had to learn simple things like how to operate the washing machine and what cleaning products to buy for the house. Even though we lived in separate houses, Sandy would come over to help with the washing and cleaning. In return, I helped her with her utility bills.

The relationship I had with my girlfriend came to an end. I could not give her the attention she wanted. To be fair to her, she did warn me she was high maintenance. I was actually relieved that our relationship ended, as I needed to deal with my sorrow and look after my son.

Time did heal me, and as time passed, I was able to return to deal with my transgender identity.

Chapter Five

Winds of Change

I let my hair grow long and continued my laser hair removal, crossdressing whenever I could. I bought a hairpiece referred to as a topper. It was not a full wig but a clip-on hairpiece that gave me more volume on top and length. I had my eyebrows waxed and trimmed. The day my topper arrived I dressed up all the way, false breast, a sexy dress, and high heels and of course my new hairpiece. I walked over to the bathroom and looked at myself in the mirror. The ugly male image was gone but instead reflecting back at me was a beautiful woman. I truly saw myself as Lisa for the first time.

Using the camera timer I took a few photos, posing in different stances. After undressing, I reverted back to my ugly self. I reviewed the pictures on my computer. I was amazed at the images I saw before me, so much so I had a strange reaction! I was actually aroused by the woman I was looking at. I kept this bizarre experience to myself. Later on, in my transition, I had mentioned this to a girlfriend. She gave me comfort in knowing that she too can be turned her own sexy images. I was happy to hear that this was a just own sexy images, that this was a just another *girl code.*

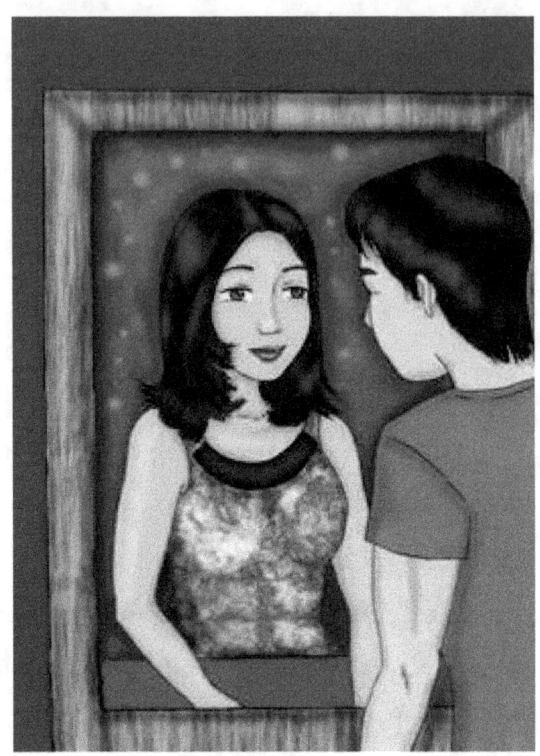

Figure 4 May 2011 Lisa appeared for the first time

A chance encounter on Friday 16th September 2011 would stop my spinning compass and set me on a new and exciting course. I met Leah, a twenty-eight-year-old exotic dancer. Destiny was at work, it did not take us long for us to forge a unique friendship "**Anam Cara**"(a soul friend, joined by the ancient and eternal way). The very next day I gave her a copy of my first book. She was eager to do a book about her life to be titled "Becoming Leah."

The first Sunday we met, we sat at her table in her two bedroom apartment. A bottle of Caribbean rum and what would become our favorite mixed with ginger ale. That night Leah opened her heart and soul to me. She too possessed two personalities. Leah was a strong, tough, resilient exotic dancer, who had to support herself and her daughter. As the night progressed, we drank more rum. She started revealing the true person hidden deep inside of her. This was Michelle a beautiful woman both inside and out. I immediately felt admiration and pity for the woman that was trapped inside of Leah. This was a trapped person that needed to be freed.

As the night wore on I was discovering more about Leah and Michelle. I strangely started discovering more of myself.

In just our second meeting over lunch at a Boston Pizza, I had mentioned to her about my transgender personality. Like her two personalities, I too had two personalities living in my body. As young as she is, by drawing a simple diagram, she was wise enough to explain to me that my two personalities were merging together to become one. It was a time in my life for my two personas to stop fighting for control of my body and mind. Lee had to accept it was time for Lisa to emerge and take over control.

Leah invited me to her friend Avaya's Halloween party, and that would open my eyes to the world of a dominatrix. Halloween was a perfect time I could dress up as a woman and go out in public.

Avaya is a beautiful, voluptuous woman of part native descent, her dark hair flows beside a beautiful, tender face. I had met her before during one of my cross dressing sessions, but her main profession is a dominatrix. Mistress Avaya is a married woman, her husband a well-endowed man from Barbados. "Damien's dick is so big. I have had many men in my life. But there is no way I could ever take such a big dick like that" Leah had explained to me while we enjoyed a pleasant lunch together at Boston Pizza the day after we had met. It was over that lunch that I had first mentioned to Leah about my GID.

The couple was both happily married and flourishing in the business of BDSM. Avaya does not offer direct sexual services, her vagina out of bounds to any client. She focused on a variety of fetishes from a dominatrix, humiliation, sub/slaves, whipping, spanking, paddles, cage play, humiliation, sissy play, role playing, forced feminization, etc...They have a dungeon in their basement equipped with an x-cross bench and all accessories hanging on the walls.

Leah recalled a time years ago when she went down to their basement. As she stepped off the last step, she noticed a figure in the dog cage in the low-lit basement. The walls were painted black adding to the darkness. Curiously she took a step closer to take a look; to her surprise, there was a man on all fours, naked staring up at her. Her head jolted backward and immediately she turned around and ran up to the living room where Avaya was casually relaxing on the sofa. Shocked and a bit bewildered Leah blurted out, "There is a man in your dog cage downstairs in your basement". Avaya casually looked up at Leah, and then looked at your watch, smiling she said: "Oh he still has 20 minutes left in the cage."

I was fortunate enough to witness a session during their annual Halloween party. That night I dressed in my black leather dress and my Steve Madden shoes, a sexy pair with a 3" heel easy to walk in. Leah helped me with my makeup; she was dressed as a Joker. The party was in full swing when finally the sub arrived at about 10pm dressed in a prisoner outfit. One of their subs arrived dressed in a prison outfit. They made him lie face down on this special spanking bench. Hand and legs strapped. Then the mistress pulled down his pants and started the play. He was spanked and told how he was a naughty boy. Everyone was able to join in. Even I spanked him. They used a paddle, riding crop, whip, etc... He was hit really hard, even to the point of some blood showing. His butt was so red. This guy is so into it that he doesn't even have a safe word. The mistress was really good at her role playing.

I was not shocked by what I saw, but a part of me enjoyed taking control and spanking the sub. I thought with my open mind I had seen it all, but this was defiantly an interesting educational experience. BDSM is not necessarily sexual, she would cater to prominent businessmen, who normally oversee or manage many employees. For a change, they want to reverse the role and be dominated or even humiliated.

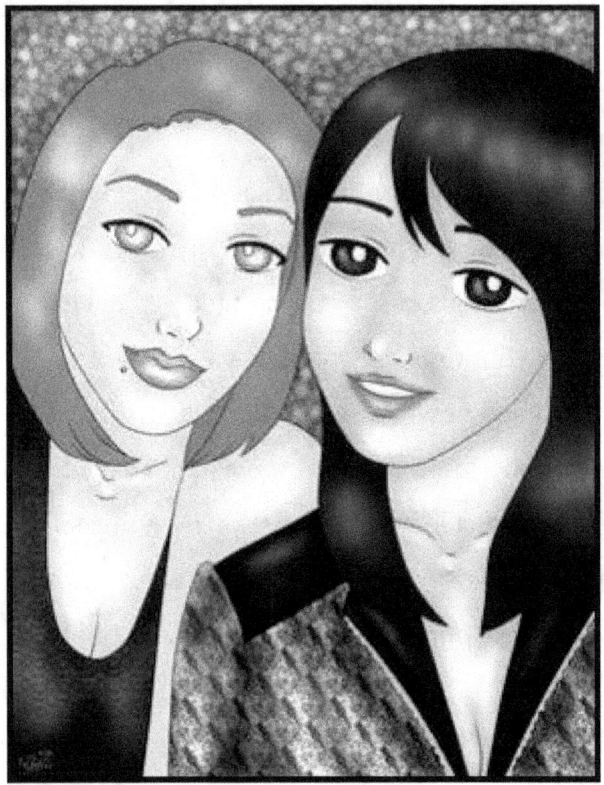

Figure 5 Leah & Lisa

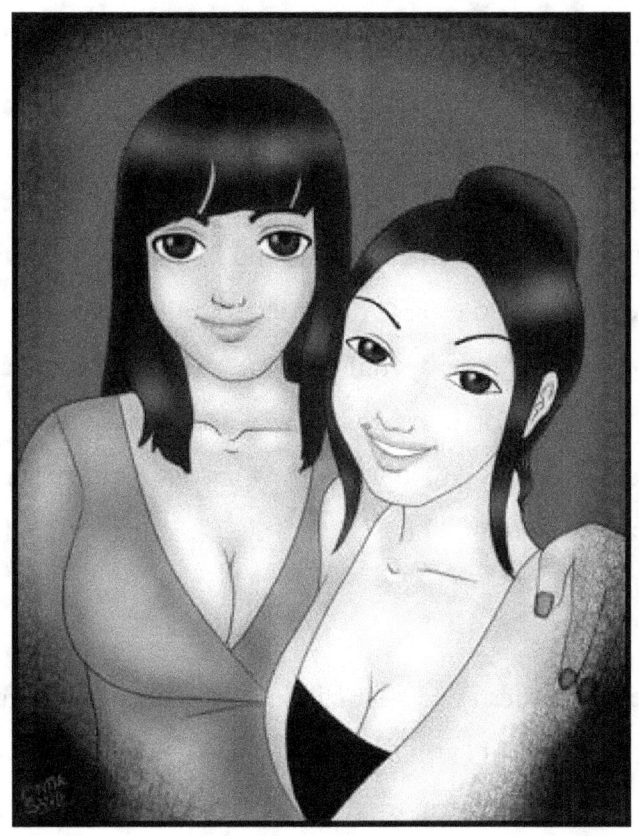

Figure 6 Lisa & Avaya

Since moving to Canada, I continued the laser beard removal on my
face, chest, and stomach. When Bret turned 18, he told me he wanted
to move out and get a place with his friends. I saw this as an
opportunity for me to start living by myself again and start pursuing
my life as Lisa. So at the age of 49, I felt I was at a point in my life
that I had to go through with this. Everything now was falling into
place. I sold the house and bought a condo in Niagara Falls.

In Dec 2011 my female Doctor M.B. who was aware of my GID for some time started prescribing me hormones after receiving the Transgender Guidelines and Protocols from Sherbourne Heath Centre. All my life I have preferred the comfort of having female Doctors. I even recall my beautiful blond haired Doctor I had at the age of five. She would crouch down in front to examine me. Her beauty and pleasant nature would put me at ease. In Curacao, I had another female Doctor, a great woman who was also aware of my GID. I had found my female Doctor in Canada. Dr. M.B. a beautiful, well educated, pleasant, honest Doctor, such a pleasure to be in her company.

That same December I had a Brazilian butt surgery using fat transfer in Miami, nobody but Leah knew I was in Miami for the week for the surgery. Before my trip to Miami, the surgeon told me what medication I needed to bring from Canada. One was for nausea to be taken the morning before the surgery; oxycodone pain killer and antibiotics. The medication I received from Canada was different brands from the ones prescribed in Miami. So that morning I took the nausea tablet in anticipation for my afternoon surgery. I found myself walking along the streets near the hotel passing time feeling so good about myself. I was so surprised at myself that I was not nervous at all for the upcoming surgery. I was just feeling so great.

That afternoon I met with the Dawn at the Surgeons office and showed her the tablets I brought with me from Canada. It was soon realized I had taken the wrong tablet in the morning. I had mistakenly taken the oxycodone that would explain why I felt so great. Anyway, no harm was done.

When I entered the room, the operating table reminded me of the table used to put condemned people to death by lethal injection. The table had a side piece sticking out where I had to lay my arm for the IV injections. It reminded me of a USA lethal injection execution table. Lying on the table, I wondered how long it would take for me to be knocked out. The next thing I remember is dreaming about my friend Leah just before waking up. Leah was the only person that knew I was doing this surgery.

The surgery went well; I had a support worker help me for the first night. An ex-flight attendant, very friendly and helpful. She had prepared food for me that day and brought it to the hotel I was staying at in Miami Beach. For a week I stayed alone at the Hotel texting Leah every day. She wished she could be with me to support and help me. The worst was that I could not sit down on my butt for a whole week. It was also very difficult and discomforting to get in and out of bed. At least the surgeon recommended I could sleep on my back, in the hope for the newly inserted fat to fill out on my hips. The beautiful Cuban front desk receptionist was very friendly and helpful to me. So before I left, I bought her a Christmas gift, the

57

perfume I would always buy for Sandy. The bottle was in the shape of a woman's body. Back home it took me another two weeks to fully recover. I did not get the hips I wanted but a good butt that even my girlfriends were envious of.

Through my Doctor, I met Vee, a transgender woman who was scheduled to have her GRS in March 2012. Meeting Vee was a great help to me, she was able to advise me on what to expect during my transitions, from dealing with family and friends to dealing with the general public. She also gave me all the important contacts needed for my transgender journey. Vee and my Doctor would later refer me to Sandy E a Psychotherapist to help me with a smooth transition. Meeting Sandy would become a very important pivotal moment in my life.

In April 2012 I had a setback. I was hoping that I would have had my Canadian Citizenship by now as it would have paved the way for me to proceed with my name change. My safety net would have been in place, no more renewing my Permanent Residency status. I would have been a proud Canadian of a country I have settled into and came to love. I had to go in front of a Citizenship Judge as I did not have the required days in Canada due to my business travel. The Judge did not rule in my favor and recommended I reapply when I have the required days. This was a major blow to me; I did have a chance to appeal. It was only after I realized I should have mentioned my transgender journey as they do have a clause for "extraordinary circumstances." Maybe it would have helped my situation. I was able to renew my expired Permanent residency Card which was valid for another five years. I then decided this should not hold me back. I need to move forward with my journey.

My sister Elizabeth and I had a special connection as we had both had to deal with the deaths' of our spouses. Finally, on19 June 2012, I plucked up the courage overwhelmed by the need to tell a family member about my GID. I sent the following email to my sister Elizabeth, with the attachment of me as Lisa

Read this first before you look at the attachment. I hope this is not too much of a shock to you, but I feel that speaking to people who are close to me helps. Do you remember when we were young, we used to change clothes with each other. I would wear yours or sleep wearing your pajamas. I remember as young as five years old, I realized that I wished I was born a girl. I used to look at you, Amy or Jean and be all envious of you knowing that you were girls and I was not. The nursery rhyme "what are little boys made of...what are little girls made of..." I used to hate and love it at the same time. All my life I have been dealing with this transgender issue. But having said that, I am only attracted to women, always have been and always will be. I know I am obsessed with women and everything about women. I've dealt this with this all my life. When I was in South

59

Africa and working at the Wild Coast, I actually went to go see a psychologist about this. I just had one session with her, at that time she asked me the question " how would you like this to turn out?" At the time I told her I wish it would just go away because that was the easiest solution to it.

I only told Sandy about this after we were separated, which was about 10 years after our marriage. She was quite shocked at first because she didn't suspect anything over the 10 years. Then she became very supportive of me. I think that is why we stayed close to each other even though our marriage was over. That is why I felt I had to be there for her too, as she gave me the support I needed. None of this had anything to do with her depression or death. I always wondered if she spoke to Bret about this. I have not yet, but have the feeling he might know. She always told me that if I needed to go pursue this further, she would be there for Bret. So that is why I had a bit of anger in dealing with her death.

When Bret turned 18, and he told me, he wants to move out and get a place with his friends. I saw this as an opportunity for me to start living by myself again and start pursuing and dealing with my transgender issue. So at the age of 49, I felt I was at a point in my life that I had to go through with this. I even went to see my Doctor, a woman that was very understanding to my situation. She started prescribing me some hormones and did all the regular blood tests. There was a time in Curacao I did take some hormones, but stopped, as it has a negative effect on the male sex drive. I felt the urgent need

60

to go through with this all the way before I got too old. But when I turned 50 I realized that there is no rush in life. Since then I have stopped with the hormones. Leah was also a big help in me discovering myself. In the process of discovering her for the new book. I found myself discovering more about myself. With her help and support, I discovered that both genders that I possess can coexist with each other. Lisa (the name I use) and Lee can coexist in harmony. I also realize there was no rush to pursue this but to try and deal with both genders.

Over the years I have been doing some cosmetic treatments. It is now fashionable for men not to be hairy. I did start laser treatment years ago, first for the beard, now I don't have to shave anymore. I also had the chest and stomach area done. With my hair growing long, my eyebrows trimmed a bit and the help of a hairpiece. I can transform very well as you can see in the photograph. When I looked at myself in the mirror, I was quite surprised at what I saw. If you remember what mom used to say to us "you are big and ugly enough to look after yourself," growing up I did think I was ugly, but when I see myself as Lisa, I see a beautiful woman. With some of the treatments that I've had like a laser or waxing, I have felt more confident with my looks, and they have even gone out in public as a woman. So at the moment I am happy switching between both genders, mostly in the privacy of my condo. But there are times the female side of me really feels so strong that I do want to actually go all the way with it. The advantage the treatments have for my male persona is that it helps me look and feel young. At my 50th the women were asking me what was my secret to me looking young. I told them it was Canada. With the cold, it is like fruit in a fridge. It will remain fresh longer, but in the sun and heat it would dry up and look old.

Through the doctor, I met a person that went through the same thing, but she went through the whole sex change operation recently. In Canada they are more acceptable to transgender people; even the Government health care covers the operation. Coming to Canada was actually a very good move for dealing with this. When I opened up to women I knew from the hairdresser, salons or shops, they were very supportive. They will always say "who are we to judge as long as it makes you happy."

So who knows what tomorrow brings? I hope you can understand my feelings as it has been very tough for me dealing with this in the earlier years. But now I accept who I am.

Love Lee

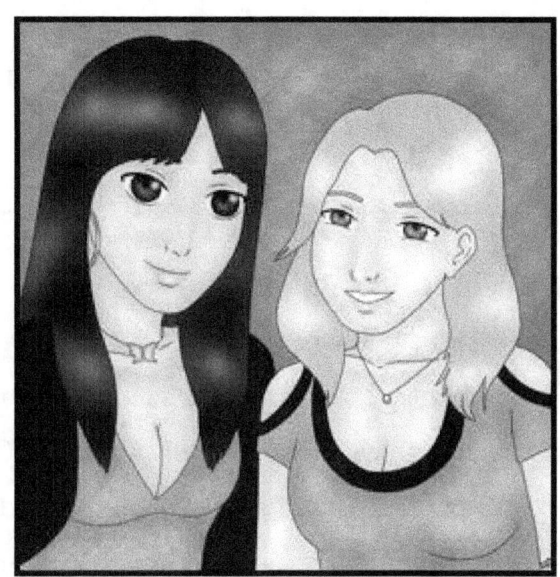

Figure 7 Lisa &Vee

Chapter Six

The Journey begins

17 July 2012, Tuesday

First Therapy Session: Vee who I had met through our Doctor recommended the Therapist she had used, Sandy E, located in Niagara Falls. At the time we met, she was waiting for GRS which was scheduled for March 2012. She was a big help in advising about my transition. I had some final reservations I had to deal with before moving forward. I had just had my neograft hair transplant done so I was not able to wear my hair piece which gives me volume on top and length on the sides and back. Dressed in my jeans I had bought from Long Tall Sally and white top, flip flops and my toenails painted.

I met Sandy at the door who led me upstairs to her study. I felt comfortable and at ease to talk to her. After I told her my story which started at the age of five I had three main points to discuss:

1. How do I tell my son? Did his mother Sandy tell him about my GID before she passed away? As she had promised me that if I needed to leave and pursue this, she would be there for Bret. Sandy advised me to talk to him about it but hold off about my planned transition. So not to overload him with too much to deal with at once.

2. One of my biggest concerns that was still confusing me. I am only attracted to women and how does this fit into my desire to become a woman. Even before I came to see Sandy, I did have an answer to this question. I had created an online profile on one of the dating websites as a transgender woman. I was pleasantly surprised at how many beautiful feminine women there were out there looking for other women. I received great support from some of the women on the site. Sandy also cleared this up for me that I should just accept that I will be part of that group of women that love women.

3. The other point was that I had started a unique relationship with a younger woman (Leah) that appeared to be more than just friends, but a relationship that was not based on sex. I did not know where this relationship was heading and if it would cause me to hold off on my transformation. She made a very important point. "Don't let a relationship hinge on your decision on your transformation. If you do decide to proceed with that relationship, if a valid one, will still be there for you." She also advised me to cautiously speak to Leah about this. I did do this in a cautious way and, I realized that Sandy had made a very valid point. The relationship with Leah is what it is, a deeper friendship that we are both lucky to have.

Sandy also pointed out two good points: That I have been preparing this transformation all my life and that I should trust my gut feelings. I have to say after days of deep thought and processing all of the above; I now saw myself as a small boat in a canal drifting at ease. I did not have to use any power as I had the gentle flow of water to propel me along the journey I so desired to venture down. I found myself preparing what I needed to do, like legally changing my name; inquiring how to proceed with my Canadian citizenship; ending of my business trips to Curacao, and my final trip to see my parents. Doing all of this without hesitation or question.

I regard July 17 as a very important date, as it paved the way for me to move forward with my journey. My final hurdles fell down, all except one, the most important one of all, my son. 17 is also my lucky roulette number, and as Sandy pointed out to me, add the 1 and 7 together you get 8 which is the sign for infinity. I searched it up on the Internet and found an even more interesting meaning of the number 8: it represents extrovert, strength and is the highest feminine number. *Reference Numerology by Joanne Sacred Scribes.*

July 26, 2012, Thursday
Laser & Filler: This was the first time I visited Niagara Skin Institute as Lisa. I had my first underarm laser removal and Restylane filler injections around the mouth and nose area.

August 9, 2012, Thursday

Tarot Card reading: My friend Nancy read my Tarot cards with a 3 card deal. Past, present & future. This is how it was read: Past: I had success and was a hard worker (all true); Present: I am dealing with internal conflict, but my head is clear (all true); the final card about my future was turned over. As a believer in my reading, I knew what card was going to appear! It was the Death Card, which does not have to mean death but rebirth (all so true with the ending of Lee and the rebirth of Lisa). I have had readings done before in the past, but none of them had anything in relation to my transgender issue.

August 15, 2012, Wednesday

Cosmetic Surgeon trip: I was able to get an American Express credit card in the name of Lisa Alexander. I had applied for an additional card under my account. I just told the woman the truth that I was transgendering and needed a credit card for when I am out as Lisa. All I needed was to give her a name and birth date. I told the truth about Lisa's age (maybe I should have lied as most women would do?)

It was a great feeling to be able to book hotel rooms in Lisa's name using the credit card and be greeted at the reception at the Fairmont Royal York Hotel as Lisa. My friend Nancy accompanied me on this trip as she had a friend in Toronto she could see. Even on the phone in the room the operator or receptionist would address me as Ma'am. Oh, that felt so good.

Later that evening Nancy and I went for a few drinks at a bar in the mall connected to the Hotel. We were greeted and served by a friendly barmaid of Italian decent. She commented, "You ladies are all dressed up, are you going out?" I explained to her about my cosmetic consultation and was just out for the night. I was dressed in a sexy, elegant black and white dress that I had purchased at Sam's Club across the border and wearing my Guess 3"slip on heels.

After a few Coors Lights, I felt the need to go pee. As I walked around the bar on the smooth wooden floor, I felt my left heel start to slip. Quickly I grabbed onto the high cocktail table to stop my slip. The plate on the table went flying into the air crashing down on the floor breaking into a few pieces; the table did not help as it was not sturdy. Before I knew it, I landed on my butt. Luckily for me, I had my new sexy Brazilian butt to cushion the landing. The Barmaid was quick to come out from behind the bar to help. I stood up smiled to contain myself. Luckily the bar was empty at that time, so it was not too much of an embarrassment for me. Headed straight to the Ladies bathroom, remembering to sit down and pee. It might sound like an easy task at hand, but for a male body to sit down to pee; your brain is telling you that you are sitting down for number two. When I returned to the bar unscathed, Nancy was quick to console me, "You have to get used to walking in those heels, I myself have slipped like you a few times, so don't worry about it girl". The barmaid was apologetic explaining that the floor had just been waxed and polished. "Oh well, shit happens." I thought it had to happen sooner or later. That day was a quick lesson I learned about the heels, yes they do make me feel sexy and look good. Not good for long walks around the mall.

Another lesson I soon realized that I had to adjust to being seen and accepted as a woman. Generally being a polite person stepping back and letting other people go before me through doors or the escalator. Men would courteously allow me to go first. I had to say to myself, "Remember you are a woman now, and there are gentlemen out there."

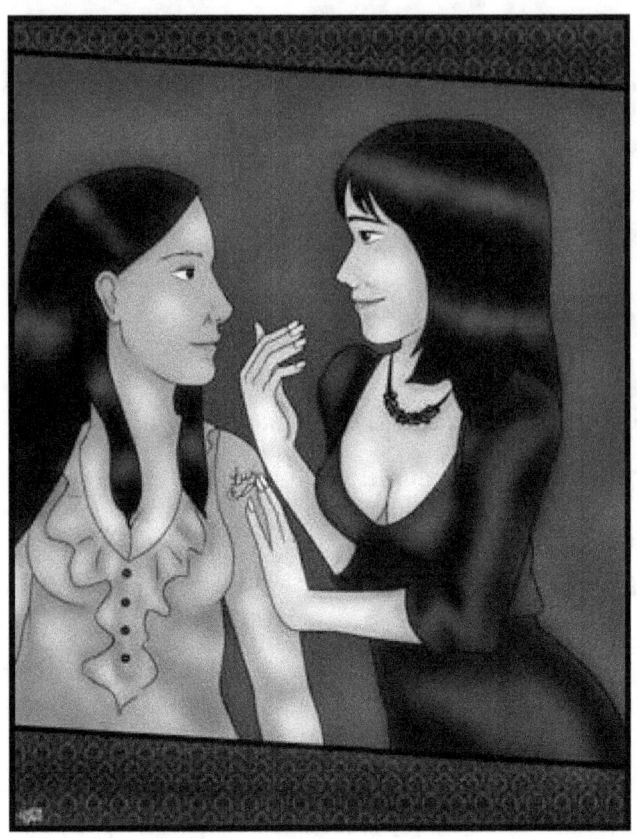

Figure 8 Nancy & Lisa

August 16, 2012, Thursday

Consultation With Dr. Martin Jugenburg .

I was up earlier than expected so Nancy and I had enough time for a quick breakfast in the coffee shop downstairs. I told her about a strange dream I had that night before. I had a dream about my late wife Sandy who supported me with my transgender quest. She had promised me, "I will be there for our son if I needed to go deal with your transformation." But after her passing, this was never possible. I could not remember what Sandy and I had spoken about. Nancy commented to me that Sandy came to me in my dream for support. This was a comforting thought, Sandy even though not here in person, but in spirit was here with me to support me.

At first, my consultation with the surgeon did not go the way I intended. I was there to see him about a possible hip enhancement surgery. I was informed that I did not have enough fat to do a fat transfer to my hips. As I had recently had liposuction in Miami and the fat transferred to my butt known as the Brazilian Butt surgery. He informed me that it normally takes up to a year for the body to fully heal from liposuction, so even if I did have enough fat, it would not be recommended to do so again within a year. I have to say it did make me feel good knowing that the stomach did not have as much fat as I did in the previous year. He did not recommend hip implants and suggested I let the hormones do the work of naturally doing the fat transfer. With hip implants, it will look good when I stand up, but not so good when I sit down.

We then discussed the possibility of breast implants. The thought of me having breasts as early as Jan or Feb 2013, excited me immensely. I was surprised to learn that with the recommended Saline breast implants for the male body and my chest size, I could even go up to a size D breast. Normally breast implants are measured by cc, not cup size. With my body, I could go as much as 800cc. I left his office so happy and excited knowing that the money I had planned for my hips could go towards obtaining a C - D breast size. Bringing me one step closer to becoming the woman I want to be. Obtaining natural looking breasts as opposed to the silicone breast forms I use will resolve two major objectives: 1. to look and feel more like a natural woman; 2. I would be able to buy dresses or tops I normally could not wear before due to the breast forms. I could finally show some cleavage.

On our way back to Niagara I explained one day to Nancy that as a woman I never know what to do with my arms when walking or just standing around. I was surprised to hear from her that she as a woman had the exact same problem. She did not know if she should just hang them loose by her sides or keep them above the waist. We both agreed we felt better with something in our hand like a cell phone or purse.

August 18, 2012, Saturday

Informing Liz: On my return to the Falls I had the urgent desire to go meet with Sandy's cousin Liz and introduce her to Lisa. As Lee, I was to meet her at the Latina night at "The Bank" in the Falls. I told her I have something to talk to her about that might shock her, but not to worry it was not in any bad way. I texted her using my Lisa phone telling her I was a friend of Lee and will meet up with her and Lee.

I arrived as Lisa and texted her that I was in the bar. As I entered, I opened my bag to pay but was quickly informed that ladies did not have to pay. "Hey being a lady does have its benefits," I thought. She replied that she would be there in five minutes. I sat in an empty section of the bar and ordered a Coors light. Half way through the beer she arrived she stood right next to me and texted Lisa, "Where are you?" She heard my Lisa phone ping and knew it was me. Sandy had apparently told her about my crossdressing. She turned around and greeted me as Lee. She was so happy I opened up to her as she spoke to me about the business that Sandy and I were going to open. Offering a safe place for crossdressers where men can go and be transformed into a beautiful woman for an hour or so.

It is said that one in four men suffer from this transgender issue or have the desire to crossdress. Liz had wanted to approach me over the past two years since Sandy's death but did not know how to approach me about this. In the meantime, she had studied as a beautician and was now ready to continue the dream that Sandy and I had. Meeting her as Lisa has brought us closer together which was once a distanced relationship. A few days later she paid me a visit at my condo and helped me with some makeup tips.

August 21, 2012, Tuesday

Laser Hair removal: I had an appointment with Emily at Laser Center for spot treatment for my chest and stomach area. In the past, I have done facial hair removal and face rejuvenation with Emily. The beard laser hair removal was a continuation of treatment I had started years ago in Fort Lauderdale. I have come a long way from heavy beard growth to a smooth facial skin. Even women would comment on my smooth skin. The facial rejuvenation which consisted of five treatments spread over four-week intervals. This was to remove sun damaged dark spots on my face. I had a distinctive dark spot on my right cheek that I was so happy to see it fade away. I had told Emily that the reason for all these treatments was for transgender reasons.

The night before Liz had done a great job on my eye makeup. I was able to sleep with the makeup without causing any smudges. So it was time for me to introduce Emily to Lisa. I arrived dressed in my pink top with a black skirt, and my Las Vegas feminine flip flops. "Hi there you look good," she said with her beautiful smile. I asked how she recognized me as I was hoping to surprise her. I was her only appointment that morning so she knew I was coming.

August 23, 2012, Thursday

Laser hair removal& Shopping: I took advantage of the special that Niagara Skin Institute had, 50% off any treatment if you purchase a package of 6. I decided on a full leg and underarm which cost me a total of $1,169.55 which would have normally cost me $2339.10. Totally worth it knowing that my legs and underarms will be hairless and no need to shave or wax anymore. I did have one underarm treatment 4 weeks ago; the pain was tolerable, in fact, less pain than waxing. Caroline, the friendly, beautiful receptionist, had advised me to take a Tylenol before to help deal with the pain. She told me with her being that of Italian descent, unfortunately, she inherited being hairy, it was painful for her. She would rather tolerate pain getting a tattoo done than laser. After starting laser hair removal on the face with the older painful lasers, I have learned to tolerate the pain. Knowing well it will bring about the results I so desire, to be more feminine. As they say: "No pain no gain."

I was dressed in my zebra top I had purchased from Giant Tiger for just $8 and my black skirt which is loose around the hips. Even though it only cost $8, it gave me a sexy, sophisticated business woman look. As noted by my friends; Nancy & Leah, when I wore the same outfit before. I started getting used to going around in my feminine flip flops, after realizing heels make me feel sexy, but not good for walking around. Caroline led me to the room and told me to remove my skirt, lie down and place the towel over my lap. Jill, the

75

pretty tall blonde knocked at the door before entering. The pain was not so bad, I have had worse, and unlike Caroline, this was far less painful than getting my tattoos. That day I decided to do the package for the bikini area.

I left their office thrilled at the idea I am taking one more step to becoming who I really want to be. It was time to treat myself as Lisa. So I drove over to Tango which was just down the street from the Laser center. It was there that I met Susan who was so helpful. I told her I was transgendering to a woman and have not developed hips yet. So needed a dress and skirt that were not too clingy and looser around the hips. I had previously purchased a black and white dress from them, which was on a sale for $44. Perfect for me, size 18, it was black on top and zebra design on the bottom. Below the bust line it flared out giving me the impression I had wide hips. I found a similar blue colorful dress which was a perfect fit and looks. Susan showed me a similar dress, this one was a colorful dress with a beautiful hint of Turkish blue. It was pleasurable for me to be able to try on female clothes before buying them.

In the past, I would buy from shops and the Internet and only get to try them on at home. Most times it worked out other times a complete disaster. They either did not fit me or were nor suited to my body.

I went into the dressing room, closed the curtain excited at been able to play dress up. I placed the dress over my head; it was an easy fit with stretchy material. As the dress fell dropped down over my body, I looked into the mirror. "God this is perfect, I love it, no matter what price it is, I have to have it," I thought. It was the perfect fit and look for me. I walked out of the changing room; Susan was standing there with some skirts for me to tray on. She too loved it and as a bonus, it came with a short black jacket. Susan mentioned that the jacket can go with other clothes.

I tried on the first skirt, it was a no go, but the elegant black one was just perfect for me. Both items I had to have. Susan tried to get me to try on some other dresses or skirts, but I was on a budget. I walked out of Tango with $188 less in my bank account for the two items. I left a very happy woman. "Lisa deserves to look classy and sexy."

August 28, 2012,Tuesday

One hour session with Sandy: Before I went to my 6pm appointment with Sandy I stopped into Tropical Nails to have a pedicure and manicure. It is a good feeling walking in and being accepted as a woman, nobody staring at you, knowing my try identity. I decided on dark purple for my nails, a change from my new favorite color "hot pink" thanks to Leah's suggestion.

When I arrived, Sandy complimented me on my dress. The colorful blue dress I had purchased at Tango. I informed her about my plan to move forward, listing my timeline and some points of interest. The two main points for my visit was

1. I will need a letter for CAMH showing that I did have some therapy and did appear in the female form. Dr. Bertola has sent off the referral to CAMH. This is an important step to start the one-year wait till GRS. They have to do an assessment to decide if I am ready for GRS.

2. My son, this is the most difficult obstacle I must still deal with. I explained I have been dropping hints to Bret. I told him that I will end my trips to Curacao and after that, I might disappear from existence to deal with what I have to do. When the time comes, I will explain to him it is a one year trial for me to live as a woman. Sandy suggested she can help talk to him, and I should tell him that I need him to see Sandy, for me. I think this is a very good idea as she said she has a way of talking to teenagers.

There was a third point I wanted to talk about. The opportunity to do the documentary, I explained to Sandy I am all for it. She sent me an email and cc to Kirstin. That night I stayed up till 1am excited by the opportunity to tell my story, I started writing down my timeline and points of interest. I sent Kristin an email attaching my Timeline/points of interest; My Tattoo story; Letter to sister explaining my GID.

The next day I was ecstatic to read Kristin's reply

"Lisa! Wow, what an opportunity you have given me- to help show the world something that I am a strong advocate for- to always be true to who you are.

I've read a bit of your story, and I'm seeing the pieces turn into a very interesting and captivating story. I am putting feelers out to friends and coworkers who I think would be right to work on your journey movie.

Here's what I'd like to do next if you are up for it- firstly, do not tell me any more until we see each other! What I'd like to do is sit down with you perhaps with a voice recorder or maybe with my camera- maybe both- and capture some of your stories. A screen test, so to speak, so that we have something to work with long term, and I can show potential key creatives - look, this is Lisa. This is her story. Look what we can do to show her story."

August 29, 2012, Wednesday

Electrolysis: At 9:30 I arrived at Brenda's house five minutes earlier and parked in her double driveway. Her door is normally unlocked, so I entered took off my flip flops. A Canadian tradition I have become custom to, removing your shoes when entering a person's house. This custom must have started from the winter months so that you don't bring in all the snow into the house. I have to say it does keep all the houses cleaner. Dressed as Lisa in a dress this was the first time Brenda would see me in my feminine form. Like other women that do my laser and waxing, I did inform her about my upcoming changes. Every time I opened the basement door, she would hear you and greet you by telling you to come down. "Be prepared for a surprise" I called out to her. As I walked into her view, I could see her pleasant surprise as I walked into the electrolysis room. I could see she was lost for words, almost dumbfounded. Finally, she turned around to me shaking her head. "Looking at you now, I just can't imagine you as a man!" I smiled knowing well these kinds of compliments were a great boost to my self-esteem. She then proceeded to do my thirty-minute session, taking care of the few white facial hairs I have that the laser treatments are unable to eliminate. The laser works well on dark hairs on fair skin, but unfortunately, lasers are not effective on white hairs. Wow, being a brunette does have its advantages over the blonds.

August 31, 2012, Friday

Meeting & Screen test. I was excited by the opportunity to meet Kristin and talk about the possibility of doing a documentary about my upcoming journey. In the morning I had to go to St Catharines to do my vending and to the Walk-In Clinic to pick up a referral letter from Dr. Bertola, which my insurance required to cover the Therapy sessions with Sandy. I had to be back in the falls by 3pm to prepare for the 4pm meeting as I had to be in male form to do my vending and meet up with my son. I was running late as I had to pass by Gisela, a beautiful Venezuelan woman that does my waxing and sugaring. I had to have my eyebrows done so that I could look the best for the camera.

I arrived back home way behind schedule only giving me ten minutes to shower, do my makeup and get dressed. It was a rush, but I managed to do a fair job on my makeup. I arrived on time at Sandy's house which is not too far from my home. Kristin is Sandy's daughter who just finished film school but already had five movies to her credit as an actress. Her new focus was to produce movies. So my transition journey was a great opportunity for her.

The idea of the meeting was to be a casual conversation that would be recorded on Camera and a voice recorder, with the possibility it may be used as a screen test. She had the camera set up in her mom's study where her Therapy sessions take place. I sat in the comfortable lounge chair facing the camera. Kristin clipped on the microphone followed by some sound tests. I was pleasantly surprised and taken back by her comment as she peered at the camera LCD display to focus, "You look very good on camera."

I have never looked good on camera as a male, there are only a few photos taken of me that I have actually liked.

I did my introduction "Hi I'm Lisa, a transgender person, and this is my story." I proceeded to tell her my story starting from when I was five years old to present day. She then followed up by asking me a few questions. She commented at the end that she felt a strong connection when she could relate to my description of how I felt growing up as a boy and would see girls in a bathing suit or leotard. I would see the smooth flatness between their legs and have the feeling that I can only describe as a homesickness feeling. She related to this as she knows very well the gut-wrenching feeling of homesickness. The meeting was supposed to be about thirty minutes without any time limit but went on for about two hours. I left feeling happy that I am able to tell my story to help others who have transgender issues and to educate people about transgender people. We are not to be feared, humiliated or made fun of. All we ask is accept us for who we are.

Later that night I spoke to Liz about my meeting, she was so excited for me to have this opportunity. She then told me something that on one hand was comforting, and on the other, a bit hurtful. Sometimes it is better not to hear certain comments. When I had left her after meeting her that night in the club dressed as Lisa. The man at the door was laughing about something. When Liz questioned him, he explained that it was funny that he did not charge me to enter knowing well that I was actually a man. It did bother me at first, what was my giveaway? My small hips or was it just that my voice was not feminine enough. After a while I thought about it, that my journey will not be easy, there will be bumps in the road, and I must just keep my head up and continue my journey forward. The comforting part is that she told me that she is not going to associate herself with the people from that business as they have no part in her life with ignorant attitudes like that. As I said before, why can't people just accept us as a person, why do we have to be judged by our gender or the way we look or dress?

3 September 2012, Monday

Vee: I was excited to receive the text that she was in the Niagara area and was able to visit. Vee had done the full transition from male to female, undergoing gender reassignment surgery in March 2012. She was an inspiration and gave me great advice and support for my transgender quest. She was a true friend and inspiration to others. I was anxious to see her and hear how she felt after the final step in becoming a full woman. There has been a major advancement in GRS, with results so good that if a transgender woman went to a doctor and was inspected below, the Doctor would assume it was a natural vagina.

When she arrived, we sat down in my lounge with the aloe vera drink she and I both enjoyed, which is both tasty and very good for you. I was dressed as Lisa but did not bother to put in my breast forms. I updated her on my decision to proceed with my Therapy session with Sandy, which I thanked her for referring her to me. But enough about me, I wanted to know how it went with her surgery.

At this point, five months after the surgery she had totally healed. She felt now that her body was right and finally comfortable with her present body. She did not miss her penis. I told her I cannot imagine the feeling of finally having all male parts removed and replaced with female genitalia. I was fortunate enough for her to show me the results.

"Do you want to see the results, are you comfortable to look?" she asked.

Containing my enthusiasm, I said, "Sure I would love to see it if you are comfortable with showing me."

She got up and moved over to the dining room table as there was lighter there. She undid the top button on her denim shorts, unzipped and pulled the shorts to just above her knees. She then proceeded to carefully pull down her white panties which contained a pad.

"I have to use pads" she explained.

"Is that for the discharge from the wounds?" I asked

"No, it is for urine drainage, as the muscle or valve that controls the bladder has to still strengthen. When I told a female friend about this, she smiled and said '*welcome to being a woman*."

I was absolutely amazed at the results. I was not looking at a fake or reconstructed vagina, but a naturally looking vagina. Her pubic hair did cover the small scars that once were the base of her penis. But wow? She had the female slit. It took me back to the moments growing up when I would look at girls' flatness between the legs and have that gut wrenching homesickness feeling, that that is how I should be between my legs. "God I want one of those" was my immediate thought.

Feeling even more reassured by the advancement of GRS, she explained to me that she had to dilate her new vagina daily so that it does not close up. They gave her sizes 1-4 dilators, so the idea is to start with the smaller one first and over the weeks or months move up in size. She would have to lubricate them and insert them for a while. I asked if she had feeling inside which she replied: "Yes and it is a joy to do."

5 September 2102, Wednesday

Appeal: Even though the sixty-day appeal period had passed for me to register an appeal about the negative decision on the citizenship. I decided to send a letter anyway for peace of mind. So I sent a letter to the Federal Court of Canada and sent a copy to the Judge that had interviewed me. In the letter I received, he wrote in his decision he stated that there were inadequate circumstances of special and unusual hardship. l wrote the following portion in my letter :

"I do realize that I am late in filing an appeal for my Canadian Citizenship application which meant so much to me personally. I held back on telling the Judge about a very personal and confidential matter. I did not feel comfortable mentioning this very personal matter to the judge at the time. I was hoping that my

citizenship would have been approved so that I could proceed on my transgender journey to becoming a woman. I know and accept that it is too late to mention this. But for peace of mind, I would like to know if my GID (gender identity disorder) that I struggled with all my life, constitutes as a "circumstances of special and unusual hardship." I am now ready to start my transgender journey, legally changing my name and making an adjustment to my career and business. At the interview with the Judge, I did pass the English and Canadian knowledge test.

6 September 2012, Thursday

Informing Vee: She was number five on my list. This was a list of female friends that would form part of my inner circle. We were to meet over a few drinks on the patio of the Regency where she now worked, today was her day off. I had prepared her that I had something both shocking and exciting to tell her.

Vee was the first person I had met at the Sunset bar that would become my temporary local pub. She showed such great hospitality and friendliness towards me. Over the month of being new to the Falls, I would enjoy the times when she was on duty, serving me my favorite Beer 'Shandy' (before pouring the beer into the glass, you would pour a bit of Sprite) a refreshing way to drink a beer. The other favorite she would prepare for me was their specialty, homemade hamburgers. She would prepare it just the way I liked it, fried onions, bacon, cheese, tomato briefly fried and no lettuce. I would call in advance for the burger so that when I arrived I would soon be served the burger, ice cold beer and her friendly greeting. She had read my first book "Putas of the Caribbean" which she thoroughly enjoyed; this also opened us to have open and frank conversations.

On the way driving to the Regency, I felt a bit nervous, not knowing how she was going to react to what I had to tell her. I arrived a few minutes before her, so I ordered a Coors light and sat on the patio to await her. As I saw her pull up in her black sedan, I thought, "This is it; I have to go through with it."

"Well, I will now test how open you are and how your shock absorbers are." I opened the conversation with. To my pleasant surprise, she was not too shocked and was so acceptable even though she said she might not agree with my decision to go through the transformation. I was so thrilled by her support and willingness to be there for me as a friend. Once again I thought how fortunate I was, I now have five compassionate and beautiful women that will be there to support me. On the way home I received a text from her, that was so touching and made me feel special.

"TY so much for revealing your innermost secrets with me ..it will Never change our friendship, and I am very flattered that u chose me to tell,cheers."

7 September 2012, Friday

CAMH letter& Accident: The big brown unmarked envelope arrived, as soon as I opened it I realized it was from CAMH. I immediately thought about what Kirstin had told me. If you receive an important letter, call us so that they can have a film crew on the scene to film me opening it. At this moment nothing had been discussed or finalized about making the documentary.

I decided to record me discussing the contents, after my quick Friday vending run. I would do some of the good locations so that I would have less to do on the following Monday.

My day was marked by a fender bender I had with an old lady. I was turning into the parking of one of my locations and had to make a sudden stop. They had repairs done to the parking area and had construction cones blocking the middle of the parking area. My car was still partly on the road so I reserved back a bit so that I could drive around the cone. All I heard was a scrape. I thought that I had scraped the bottom of my car on the curb. But soon realized it was an old lady that had scratched my car and had stopped a few meters away from the incident. I hoped this could be resolved without insurance claims as it will result in higher premiums.

I had to fill in the Transgender questionnaire and write a life story about my transgender identity. I was also suggested but not mandatory to send a photo so that they can put a face to the questionnaire. That night I did not waste time. I called Sandy for a bit of advice, she said I must tell her that she is there to support me and can supply any information they at CAMH require. Unfortunately, Transgender conditions still fall under "mental health" CAMH stands for Centre for Addiction and Mental Health. I completed the questionnaire and wrote a three-page story about Transgender history to date.

8 September 2012, Saturday

CAMH Mailing: Once again I set up my camera in video mode and recorded me showing the two important documents that were ready to be mailed. I inserted the papers into the pre-addressed CAMH envelope which also had my return address on the top left-hand corner. I soon left to mail the envelope registered mail.

9 September 2012

D-Day: At the end of the night I sat at my computer to write a letter to Elizabeth. Before leaving the lounge, I got Bret to stand up, and we hugged. Something we have not done in a while since he had not slept over in a while. With his full-time work schedule, I had to be fair with him to allow time with his friends. At least we had that lunch together on a Saturday or Sunday. But tonight he was sleeping over as we had to cross the Border so that we can get the green USA I-94W Visa Waiver document in our passports. This way when we cross over to Buffalo airport for our flights to South Africa, we would have a quicker process through American immigration.

I sat at the computer wrote and emailed Elizabeth the following letter:

Well, tonight I sat down with Bret. I did pray a lot the day before that today it would go well. A good saying I heard from a man in the Sunset Bar "you can have faith without having religion" Meaning that I don't go to Church every Sunday, but I do have the faith. Well, I have to thank God and good Canadian weed as It went better than he ever expected.

We sat on my patio smoking the joint together, with the beautiful Niagara scenery before us. I did not have to tell him in so many words what I will be doing. He replied he knew what I was planning to do. Sandy must have prepared him for this day and told him that this day would come. I have a lot to thank Sandy for preparing Bret for defining a moment in time. I was prepared for the worst reaction, but fortunately, the worst did not come. He did not say much, but I knew from his calm manner that he did have some acceptance. When there was silence after I had spoken, I would test the tension between us by passing the joint or making a comment about it. He reacted in business, as usual, a pleasant, warm and friendly chemistry that we share as father and son. I did apologize for my actions and know what effect they will have on his life. He lost a mother and is about to lose a father. I explained even if my outer image might change, I will always be the same person.

I asked if I should give up my vending route in St Catharines in respect for him. He said it was up to me as not everyone in St Catharines' will know. We did find a compromise which I had thought of at the last session I had with Sandy. I should change my car so that when Lisa takes over the vending route she will have a different car. My car sticks out like a sore thumb; it is a ford Escape copper color. I got it for a real good price with low mileage. The young salesman said to me the day before I bought it "you will grow to love the color." Well, I have to say I did grow to love the sporty looking color that would sometimes appear to be a dull orange shade.

I will let you know further how things progress. By the way, weed is not legal but decriminalized and accepted by most people.

If you think that Jean is at a good stage, you can pass this onto her.

Love Lee

13 September 2012, Thursday

Beautiful One visit. Nancy accompanied me to Mississauga after she finished work at the nursing home at 1:30pm. I picked her up at the nursing home and headed out to Mississauga. Beautiful One Clinic had done my neograft hair transplant about two months ago. The Doctor wanted to do a follow-up checkup, and I wanted to enquire about the Laser Lipolysis to remove my double chin. We

91

arrived about an hour earlier but at least they were able to schedule me in earlier. I had informed them that I will be visiting as Lisa, the Doctor was aware of my transgender intensions.

I had to use the bathroom, so I picked up the key at reception and headed off to the ladies toilet. I entered the stall, now becoming custom to sit down and pee. Out of habit, I would always place toilet paper on the seat before sitting down. This was a hygienic habit I had picked up a long time as a male, obviously when doing number two in a public restroom. I closed the door sat down on the paper-covered seat; normally three slips did the job. This bathroom trip was a new experience for me as this was the first public ladies bathroom I had visited that had graffiti on the back of the door and words. I sat down thinking 'this is going to be some juicy graffiti to read. Unlike in male toilets that are full of sexual or crude comments. These female comments had more to do with relationships than sex. It was a very interesting observation noting how the two genders express themselves in different ways.

After I had removed my top hair piece, the Doctor examined the new hair growth. He commented it was healing well, but I must still wait six weeks before seeing the new growth. We then discussed the options to remove my double chin that was so noticeable in photos when I was looking down. I did not have too much fat but loose skin. He recommended the laser Lipolysis a procedure that eliminates the fat by laser and tightens the loose skin. The procedure would take

92

about one and a half hours, followed by wearing a bandage around the head and chin for three days. He quoted me $2,500 for the procedure. Something I had learned from my mother and used very successfully over the years. Don't be afraid to ask for a discount. You would be surprised at how many times you will receive a discount just for asking. He was prepared to knock off 10% dropping the price to $2250. Not a bad deal as long as the results will be good, as another clinic in Toronto had quoted me $4,000 via email.

14 September 2012, Friday

Nancy's Birthday: Nancy slept over Thursday and Friday so that she could hang out with me as Lisa. She had missed Lisa as we had not seen each other for a while. We did at Leah's' daughter's birthday a few days before, but I was as Lee. She commented to me that I am happier and open as Lisa. She defiantly prefers the company of Lisa over Lee.

We decided to stay in at my condo to celebrate her birthday. Three of her friends turned up and with the music playing and the drinks flowing, we had a great time. The Falls even had a fireworks display for her birthday. *Lol*, every Friday in the summer they have fireworks which can be viewed for my condo patio. Later that night I found myself playing Therapist with the thirty something couple that was here at the party. With both of them telling me about their relationship problems. I guess people are drawn to me to talk about their own problems as they see me as a person who has the courage to overcome a major "*disorder*."

18 September 2012, Tuesday

The Good the bad & Ugly: In the morning I received a reply letter from the Federal Court as I was enquiring about the appeal on the Citizen Judge on my application. I was denied the citizenship as I was short the required time in Canada due to lost time from my business travel. By the end of the year, I can reapply as I will have the required days in Canada. In the Judge's ruling, he mentioned I did not have "*circumstances of special and unusual hardship*" I was curious to know if my **Gender Identity Disorder** would have qualified as "special hardships." Anyway, I did pass the 60 day appeal period deadline. If I had to pursue the appeal, I would have to have to get legal counsel. Canada Citizenship & Immigration did confirm by phone that my transgender transition will not have a negative effect on my new application. The good news is that my new application will be under Lisa.

I found an interesting opportunity on Kijiji for a small vending business for sale. The eight vending machines located in Hotels in Niagara-On-The-Lake. I immediately called and had a good conversation with the gentleman who is selling the business. The reason for the sale was due to his illness. This could be a big help in replacement income for next year. I explained to him that for personal medical reasons I am interested in his business as I have to give up my consulting travel. We set up a meeting on Thursday at one of the locations.

While I was on the phone with him, I had a private number call on my cell phone. When I checked my voice message, I realized it was a very important call from CAMH confirming that they received my questionnaire. The lady on the phone named "Sandy" did say that it will take up to 12 months before my assessment. I had mentioned before to my Therapist Sandy that every Sandy I have ever met, I had a special connection with them. This was a good sign. Sandy informed me that I can send any important documents in the meantime. This was my legal name change and testimonials that I am now living in the gender of my choice. I asked her if the one year waiting period before having GRS would start only once I have my first assessment.

One of the requirements before having GRS is that you have to live for one year in your new gender. This way a transgender person can make the final decision if they do want to proceed. This concerned me as it would mean a total wait time of two years before having the final step. I returned the call to ask her when the year would start; she was unable to give me the answer, so she transferred my call to the Doctor that would be handling my case. Unfortunately, I received her voicemail. I was very happy to know that the psychologist was a woman, as I find it easier to speak to a woman about my transgender issues. I feel that a woman will always be more understanding about my desire to be a woman, as they will know the beautiful feeling of being a woman.

I called the Registrar General to enquire how long it will take to process the legal name change. They informed me that the legal name change will take up to 8 weeks. So I decided to proceed with the application as early as possible. Later that night I completed the application. I had to fill in my present names; new names; parents' names and to confirm that there are no pending criminal or financial claims against me.

All my happiness was dampened when I got the call from the Niagara Police about the accident. The Police officer said he would come by my place to see me. Dressed as Lisa, I had to quickly transform back to Lee as the accident was all recorded under my male persona. I hate having to do these quick changes from Lisa to Lee. I look forward to the day when my name is legally changed to Lisa so that I can remain as in the gender of my choice. I thought that they were finally coming to take my statement for the accident. But instead, the dark haired young policeman handed me a summons to appear in court as I was charged with "*failing to yield from a private driveway.*" This really upset me; I was quick to show him the photos and explained to him what actually happened. He said that I can explain this on my first court appearance which is set for 20th November. What upset me most of all was the fact that I was not given the chance to make my report on the accident. If they had received it, there was no way I would have been charged.

When he left, I called the Niagara Police department to complain and was told that I must speak to the officer that issued me the summons. He soon called back. I expressed to him that I wanted to resolve this as soon as possible, as I do not want to be stressed out. I did not tell him about the transgender journey I had just started. But instead told him I have more serious medical things to worry about, I don't need any stress like this; he explained that this always happens and that it is not as bad as it sounds. Hell yes, it is, with me in the middle of my transformation and name change, how I appear in court. That night it took me a while to fall asleep. I had to go to the courthouse in the morning and resolve this matter.

19 September 2012, Wednesday

A brighter day: I woke up determined that today will be a better day. I had the documents ready for the name change. I had to sign the application in front of a Commissioner of Oaths and to have a Guarantor's Statement from a person, like a bank manager, who has known me for over 12 months. The Guarantor's Statement is also to show that I have been an Ontario resident for longer than 12 months. My other mission was to go to the courthouse to try and resolve the accident problem.

My first stop was 71 King Street, St Catharines, the courthouse for traffic offenses. I parked my car in a pay parking lot, purchased a three-hour ticket, expecting that this could take some time. I placed the parking ticket on my dashboard and headed to the courthouse. I met the pretty blonde woman at the clerk's office and explained my situation. She explained that the 20th November date was just a first administration meeting. On that date, I can put in my plea and if a guilty plea I pay a fine. But this option comes with a burden of possibly losing driving points and an increase in insurance premium. She explained to me that I do have the right to go to the police station and make an official complaint about how the case was handled.

So the next stop was 68 Church Street, a quick five-minute walk from the courthouse. There I met the female receptionist, who gave me two options; I could first speak to the officer's sergeant when he comes on shift a night, If that fails the next option is that I can file a complaint OIPRO (Office of the independent Police review Director). Later that night I did speak to the Sergeant who was very pleasant over the phone. He did confirm to me that the officer should have taken my statement to be fair to both parties. Unfortunately, the charge has already been filed, so he recommended I plead not guilty and speak to the prosecutor to have it thrown out.

As a precautionary measure, I did go see the "Roadrunner" an office that helps you fight traffic offenses. I am still waiting on the Paralegal to call me to discuss my options.

20 September 2102, Thursday

CAMH call & Business Meeting: While I was over the border in the USA purchasing some chocolates for my business, I received a call from the Doctor from CAMH. After listening to her voice message, I immediately called her and was lucky to get her on the phone. I asked her when the one-year dates start. I was so happy to hear that it is not when I have my first assessment. I have to show proof of when I have started living in the gender of my choice. This can be done in the form of testimonials and most importantly I must send her a copy of the legal name change certificate. This way all correspondence will be done in my new legal name LISA. Her encouraging words over the phone brought a big smile to my face. The accident worries were washed away by a feeling of joy, knowing that my transgender journey will transcend any negative or bad moments.

On the way to Niagara-On-The-Lake to look at the vending opportunity, I had just one very important thing to do. I mailed off the documents to the Office of the Registrar General at the cost of

$11.70 for registered mail. Now there is no turning back, full speed ahead, in just eight weeks I will legally have a new name.

The meeting and tour of the five vending locations went well. I expressed to him that I was interested, but we had to settle on a fair price. He originally wanted $9,800 based upon his gross sales. I showed him the calculation I had done in Excel, working out what his net was based on the 35% cost of sales and 15% of the locations. He was willing to drop to $7,000, and I was looking at an offer of about $6,000. Later that night I made him a proposal that we could both get what we wanted. I offered $6,200 cash at the beginning of October, with him taking the sales money for October. This way he should get his $7,000 or possibly even more and I will pay the amount I am comfortable with. He said he will discuss it with his wife, so I await his reply.

26 September -1 October 2012

Trip to Curacao. For my second to last trip to Curacao, I used my American Airlines miles to purchase the flight, Business class all the way. As with my recent trips, I was getting tired of traveling, and the Caribbean heat was starting to get to me. What a pleasure it is to be now living in a country with four seasons. Fall was upon us, my favorite season, not too hot or cold, but fresh temperature accompanied by the beauty of the changing tree colors.

I had another mission on this trip. I was meeting my friend Terry; he would be the first male friend that I would inform about my major life changes. Terry and I go back a long way, we met each other at Sun City where I started my casino career. He encouraged me back in 1984 after just ten months working as a Slots Technician to join him and Harry on a backpacking trip to Europe. With my final cheque converted to one thousand US Dollars and the pension fund payout that paid for my air ticket to London. Later on in life when I moved to Curacao he joined me there after I was able to secure him a Slots Manager position through the same group I was working for. Harry soon joined us in Curacao. Terry and I have always remained true friend over the twenty-eight years. He was even my official photographer at my wedding in the Dominican Republic back in 1989.

Terry picked me up at the airport; he knew I had something important to tell him. He would soon know the reason why I told him I would not be able to travel as of 2013. We found a vacant table inside a bar at Wilhelminapleiin in Punda.

He commented to me, "You are keeping me in suspense."

I had to get us drinks first before I could start to tell him. I needed to have a drink in my hand as this was once again another challenge for me to reveal my true self. I could not wait for the waitress, so I picked up two ice cold Polar beers at the bar. My throat was full of emotion as I began to tell him the secret I have been carrying with me for forty-five years. I informed him of the whole story and my intentions. His first comment was that he never suspected anything, but did know that like him we both had strong love towards women. He was actually relieved as he thought I was going to tell him I had a terminal illness. He commented that he was open-minded and that twenty years ago transgender would be considered taboo, but nowadays it is more acceptable.

I was so pleased with his acceptance, a proof of true friendship. He insisted that this would not change our friendship and that I am welcome to visit him in Fort Lauderdale as Lisa. Now I had my first male friend on board in my inner circle. I did take Tammy's advice on this trip to reflect on the good times I had over the twenty-four-year history of this island. This was my island in the sun I had dreamed about when growing up in Africa. Soon I would be leaving my island in the sun for good, just one more final trip. Then my life will enter a new phase, my new life completely as Lisa. I looked forward to the day I can remain as Lisa and not switch back to my male form as I had to do for the business trip to Curacao.

5 October 2012, Friday

Niagara on the Lake meeting: I had to drive over to meet the Manager of the Hotel group where the vending machines are located. The plan was that I will take over the vending route as of 1st of November. I so wanted to go as Lisa, but they were expecting Lee. The twenty-minute drive is a beautiful scenic drive through the wine farms. Just six minutes' drive from my condo you hit the first wine farm. The meeting went well; I left with a bunch of forms I had to fill out for the Hotel group.

Back home I filled out all the forms and decided to use only my initial "L" for the first name. I spoke to the gentleman I was purchasing the Vending business from on the phone. I told him about my transgender change, the second male in ten days. He was totally cool about it , telling me that Canada was an accepting nation. Even in his full-time work industry, he had known of other transgender people making the change. He made the same comment that I stand by, "It is still you as a person; they will be dealing with," referring to the new working relationship with the hotel group. So when I emailed the forms back to the female buyer, I informed her that I was in the process of legally changing my name for transgender reasons. So Monday I will see her reaction.

6 October 2012, Saturday
Laser hair removal: I had my second appointment to do my full legs, underarms, and bikini area. But this time, there will be a new area to do. I decided to do one full "Brazilian" which includes the butt or "back door" as my sugaring woman would say. The night before, I had to delicately shave all the areas, which included the bottom part of my penis. There was no way I wanted hair inside my vagina, once the penile skin is reversed inside to create the inner

walls of my vagina. I have to say some of those parts were more sensitive, including the scrotum.

Roxanne did a great job, even knowing which areas to do without me telling her the important areas. Through all the pain I was so happy, I did it.

Fall was upon us, so after the treatment, I drove over to Tango to get some warmer clothes. Lucky for me Susan was there, she even remembered my name. I have to say the first three outfits I picked up fitted me perfectly. Looking at the mirror in the change room I could see the feminine body developing. It was the first time I was trying on long pants other than jeans. The black "Travel by Tribal" was a perfect fit and the soft material felt great as it caressed my smooth thighs. With the long sleeve, animal print top gave me the sexy business woman look. The other piece was a black Temptations sweater with a belt, perfect for those cold nights when I need to look elegant.

13-23 October 2012

South Africa: Finally the day arrived; this was my second to the last trip as Lee. This was a very important and emotional trip. I had not seen my parents and family for almost three years. This would be my last trip to South Africa and possibly the last time I will see my aging parents. My father at the time was 89 and my mother 82, which is a blessing in disguise. Even though they both now have difficulty walking or getting out of a car, they both still look good for their age. As everyone points out to me, it is a good sign of good genes for a long life.

It was a surprise visit, only my sister, and her family knew we were coming. Eighteen hours of travel each way just gave us 8 days with the family. It was to be a very emotional trip for me, but I looked at it on the positive side, quality time with my family. I dreaded that final day when I had to hug my parents possibly for the very last time. But I knew I was returning back to Canada to a happy place. A new life was ahead of me and I was fortunate to have my dear friends to support me. I could not hold back the tears as I quickly hugged my Dad and then my Mother. Like ripping off the band-aid, I prefer to say my goodbyes quickly, trying to hide my emotions, the tears streamed down my face. I did not look back as my sister, and her husband drove us to the airport.

The engines roared, and I was sucked back into my seat, as the SAA plane sped down the runway at the new Durban airport, bound for Johannesburg. Then a two-hour layover in Johannesburg, then onto the SAA airbus for the fourteen-hour flight back to New York. Connecting to Buffalo, New York followed by a thirty-minute drive over the border back to Niagara Falls. For convenience, I had parked my car at the Quality Inn near the Buffalo airport. As I sat on the plane, the long journey ahead back home all I could think of was, what a perfect time I had spending time with my family. I realized how fortunate I am to come from a family of five children, all who have lived past the age of fifty. From a group of childhood friends of seven, only two of us were still alive today. Three of my close friends not even living to see their twenty-first birthdays.

1 November 2012, Thursday

New car, New business: The night before there was a lot on my mind, thinking about the new venture I was about to embark. I took over the eight machines at Niagara-On-The-Lake hotels. That afternoon my new car would be ready. I made sure I would accommodate my son's request for me to change my car. So that his friends would not recognize me as Lisa. My copper-colored Ford Escape would stick out like a sore thumb, as my car would pull up to a place I was going. The recipients I would visit would always know that it was me by the color of my car. The used car dealer was happy to receive my bright car, as all the cars in his lot were dull colors. My good old Escape would brighten his lot. I settled for a Pontiac minivan which would help with the new vending machine business.

4 November 2012, Sunday

Lunch: I had my regular Sunday lunch with my son in St Catharines. He had recommended Boston Pizza as there was something he wanted on the menu. He ordered the chicken pasta linguini. We shared one of our favorites, spinach dip served with garlic pita bread in the shape of small pizza slices. When the waitress passed by she commented, "It must be good?" looking at the dish which we divulged in no time. For my main course, I had the starter tenderloin wrapped in bacon, a tasty dish but was not crazy about the pink sauce that came with it. The replacement chipotle sauce did the trick.

Towards the end of the meal, I said to Bret, "Now that I have the new car you know that this means my new life begins?"

"I don't want to talk about it." Was his immediate response. There was a moment of silence until I broke the silence with idle chatter. It was comforting to see our conversation soon return to normal. But my heart was hurting. I felt for him knowing that he would soon lose his father. Two and a half years ago he lost his mother, now he was about to lose not me in person but, the fatherly figure he had known for almost nineteen years.

After lunch, I dropped him off, and we said our pleasant goodbyes. It's in moments like this I question myself, not doubting the journey I have started. But I feel the pain knowing that my transformation must be tough for him. My son, who I love so much does not deserve to be put through another ordeal. The only comforting thought that comes to mind is that I know he will come through this. I saw through his silence after Sandy's death he did not want to ever speak about the death. He was okay to speak about his mother remembering past moments with her. So I am sure he will ride out the storm once again. Remembering the words he told me when I had asked him if he would see my Therapist on my behalf.

"I don't believe in Therapist, I believe in self-therapy!"

5 November 2012, Monday

Vending as Lisa: Now that I had the new car. I was able to do my vending as Lisa. The problem with honor vending is as the name states. You have to rely on people being honest and to pay for the chocolates they take. There are no coin acceptors, they can just lift off the lid to take out the chocolates and insert the coins in the money box. Part of the income goes to a certain non-profit organization I support.

So today was a new challenge, how would the locations react when I enter as Lisa to change out the boxes. To my surprise, it went well, with most people not showing any surprise. The only location was the gentleman at the Tattoo shop. He raised his eyelid in a pleasant surprise. He was a pleasant person with plenty of piercings and tattoos. I smiled and said, "Same person, new gender!" to which he responded with a nod of approval. I think most people did not even notice the difference as my hair was long, both ears pierced as Lee. So only the longer hair piece and breasts set us apart. Fall was upon us so I was dressed in my black jean which had a high waistline, black top and my low heel boots, which come up just below the knees. These boots have become my favorite and most comfortable footwear ideal for the fall and winter.

7 November 2012, Wednesday

Therapy session: I was anxious to see Sandy as I thought to update her on all recent developments in my transition. A lot had happened since my last visit. So the first thing we discussed is all the updates. There were two main points I needed to discuss with her

1. The pain that I felt thinking about my son knowing that I was now moving ahead with the new car.

2. This was a most difficult one that I had to work through. With me starting a new business I had started most of the preparation work as Lee. This was partly because of my financial and credit approvals. I had to do them as Lee. But now that I was moving ahead as Lisa, how do I approach new clients. Do I go see them as Lisa or Lee? There are advantages to both sides, if I go as Lee I can go through without having to explain myself as a transgender person or worrying what they might think of me. Once Lee has secured the business deal, then they could meet me as Lisa for future business dealings. On the other hand, if they met me as Lisa from the onset, there is no need to explain the switch from Lee to Lisa. This was a complicated issue I had to solve. As I had my first appointment with a private school to place one

of the healthy vending machines. The locator had informed the administrator that Lee will come see her. My friend Nancy had advised me the night before that I should not risk anything about business. Do what I need to do.

As Sandy has told me before that, I must trust my gut instinct. She recommended that it was okay as to play both gender roles if I felt the need to do so. She explained to me that sometimes she would go into a meeting either wearing her power suit or in feminine dress, depending on the situation. She went on to explain to me that this is normal to being a woman. If I really felt the need to go in, as Lee and felt more comfortable doing it this way, to seal the deal, I must not feel bad about doing it. My main concern was I felt that I was cheating in a way when I had to revert back to Lee to take care of things. Then I realize that's this is a year's transition period and that there will be ups and downs. So these kinds of situations will arise, and I will have to deal with them.

I then explained to her how my friends Leah had introduced me as Lisa to her daughter saying that I was Lee's sister. She said to me that this is a perfect way to deal with this with the business associates that are not close to me. Lisa will become Lee's sister to some people, to certain people if they do have their suspicions, well that is for them to deal with. Some people will believe what they need to believe.

I felt once again my superhero Sandy, had put my mind at ease. I did not have to feel bad or guilty about the fact that I had to switch between both genders to take care of business. Introducing myself as Lisa as Lee's sister was actually an easier way to put people at ease and not complicate matters. Only those close to me will know the truth about my transgender change. Another beautiful comment she made to me was, "You as Lisa are destined for greatness" her comments made me really feel great. Compliments and positive thinking are always welcome and inspiring in my life, especially during these trying times. So along with Sandy's brilliant advice and Nancy's advice I felt reassured on what I needed to do.

9 November 2012, Friday

Doctor visit: Once again free to go to St Catharines as Lisa. I went to see my Doctor for a flu shot and to hear my results from my recent blood test I did on Halloween day. The ladies at the lab were dressed in costumes, but none as a vampire as they said it might have scared the older folks.

I arrived at the receptionist's and handed over my health card and explained my situation to the pretty receptionist, she was always pleasant.

"You look great, I love your hair. I have always wondered how you would look as Lisa." the words from her were so comforting and always a treat to hear good compliments.

My blood work and blood pressure were perfect. Last year was the first time I have ever received the flu shot. Due to my regular consulting traveling I had decided to get one. So this year with my transitioning, it was worth taking it to avoid the nasty flu with all the hormones and vitamins I had to take daily. It is always a pleasure to see my Doctor. A pretty happy woman that always appears to be more beautiful every time I see her. This time, her brown hair was tied up in a ponytail.

It was decided that I could increase my hormone intake. Estrogen now at 3mg and the Spironolactone 75mg. I went next door to the pharmacy and was pleasantly greeted by the woman I was attended to before as Lee. The first time I was prescribed Estrogen, while I was waiting for them, the pharmacist came up to me and politely questioned if they were for me. As soon as I mentioned it was for transgender reasons, there was no concern. So seeing me as Lisa for the first time was so natural.

12 November 2012, Monday

Happy morning. Last week I had done area 1 as Lisa, now it was time to do area 2 out of the three areas I have. I had to pick up brochures from my printer that also had one of my honor boxes. The owner was also South African, who I had done regular business with. So I thought it was appropriate to email him my situation which read as follows:

"On a confidential personal note, so that you and your employees don't get too surprised. I am legally changing my name to Lisa Alexandra as at November for transgender reasons, hence the new cards I had ordered. Thanks, Lee"

He replied by thanking me for letting him know and said he would pass it onto the others. When I picked up the brochures. Amy, the pretty blonde woman attended to me. She remarked that the younger adults were more accepting to transgender people. On the way to the van, I met up with the owner, Brad who addressed me as Lisa. We had a very pleasant conversation about my situation. He wished me well saying that it was good that I was doing something that would make me happy.

Complicated afternoon: Lee received the call that my three new vending machines would be delivered at 3pm. At 2:30pm I received a call from the driver that he was in front of my storage. So I told him that Lisa will be there in a few minutes. The 8' x 10' storage unit was located just down the street from me, just 5 minutes away.
I arrived there shortly as Lisa of course. To my surprise, the driver was alone, with no one to help unload the machines. There was another complication, the three packages were too tall to fit through the door and at 230kg, and there was no way the two of us could maneuver them in. I asked the driver how we could resolve this, are

there no one else we can call to help. He made the call to his office to see what could be done. After closing the cell phone, he said. "They will call Lee to see what could be done."

Oh no, I thought this is going to be awkward as I heard my phone ring. I quickly answered it. It was the office asking for Lee.

"Sorry he is not available; this is Lisa can I help?"

After asking them what could be done, they explained to me that the driver can only be there for an hour. So I had to come up with a solution quickly. Soon the gentleman Shaun that had helped Lee secure the storage unit came over to see if he could help. This was awkward moment number two. Would he recognize me in my feminine role? It was comforting to know he did not recognize me. Just an hour ago I had visited my friend Victoria in the same attire. I was reassured by her comment as she looked me up and down.

"Fuck you look like a hot woman." all I could do is just smile at the compliment.

This was a moment Lisa had to resolve the situation, not Lee. Proudly to say I did come up with a solution. I instructed him to leave the machines in front of the storage unit. I would rush home and find a moving company that could help me unpack the machines and move them into my storage. This was a job that required three or four men to do. I had to move quickly as dark clouds were in the sky, the rain was coming.

Back home I found a moving company that could come help but after 5pm, the same time they lock the gates. Ok, Lee it is your turn. I quickly called Shaun.

"I heard there was a situation at the storage for the machines," I said to him. He went on to tell me (Lee) what had gone on, not knowing that it was actually me there at the storage as Lisa. He said he would keep the gate unlocked for me. I sat back in my comfortable office chair and just smiled.

"Well done Lee & Lisa you just pulled off the two personality roles." I said to myself. Sandy's advice had just proved to have worked.

16 November 212, Friday

Informing Harry: The Skype phone rang, it was Harry. We had not spoken in a while. I did inform him that I had something very confidential to tell him. Since my 50th birthday, we have both been working hard on a new concept that we came up with called LinkaPub. We had made great strides in technical breakthrough on realizing our new project. We both spent countless hours researching, finally coming up with solutions. This is how we explained it on our website.

"Our Business Philosophy
Making social networking more sociable. The goal is to link pubs worldwide. So that friends and family can sit down and have a drink with each other no matter what part of the world each person is in."

I decided today was the day I will inform him about Lisa.

"I hope you have good shock absorbers, for what I am about to tell you."

This was only the second male friend I will be informing. Once again I was filled with emotion as I explained to him my past, present, and future transgender condition. Surprisingly he told me he had just watched a documentary that very week about two women that had transgendered from female to male. His conclusion was, "Good on them for going through with it".

His first comment to me was. "I feel very touched that you chose me as a friend, confiding in me with your major life change."

I told him that I found women more understanding and acceptable to my transgender change. He responded that he thought that it should be easier for males to understand than females. He told me he will be there for me and support me.

"Now that is a true friend." Once again I thought, "Why am I so blessed to have such great friends in my life?" I emailed him the picture of me as Lisa so that he can see who my present and future self is. His only concern was, when do I start calling you Lisa. I told him not to worry until after my final trip to Curaçao. He could also call me by my other name that my close friends back in South Africa would call me "Lee." A gender neutral name I actually had preferred to than Lee. Maybe I should have started using that name with friends I had made in my Casino career.

I also discussed with him my original plan to make people think I had passed away. He too had preferred my new plan that I would tell people who were not in my inner circle. That I will be taking a one to two year sabbatical to go up north and live with the Native Americans.

Soon after we closed off the Skype call I received the following reply from my photo:

"Ok...Nice

Probably still have a thousand more questions

Taking time to get used to the idea

How do I meet up with you for a week holiday in the Caribbean for your 60th without upsetting my wife?

Does she tell her friends Harry has gone to the Caribbean for a week with Lisa....or Harry is on the phone again for an hour to Lisa? We will have to "adjust."

Mate. I am not running. I will support you, and your life change is in confidence with me.

Make sure Bret is ok at all times. He has lost his mum and now he is losing a dad.

This is probably my biggest concern is for Bret. Make sure he gets the support he needs and does not flip out."

26 November 2012 Monday

Office of the Registrar General: Returning from doing my Monday vending route. I opened the mailbox and saw the white envelope from the Office of the Registrar General. "Was this the legal name change certificate, the envelope looks too small for a certificate?" I thought. Containing my emotions, I calmly walked into my apartment placed the mail on the round glass dining room table. I had to pee, the hormones as expected made me urinate more often. Calmly I set up my HD camcorder that I had bought off EBay. I mounted the camera on my tripod and pressed record. "This is either good or bad news," I said looking at the camera as I sliced opened the envelope. I stared motionless at the purple/pink document. I could not hold back the tears. Finally, it had arrived:

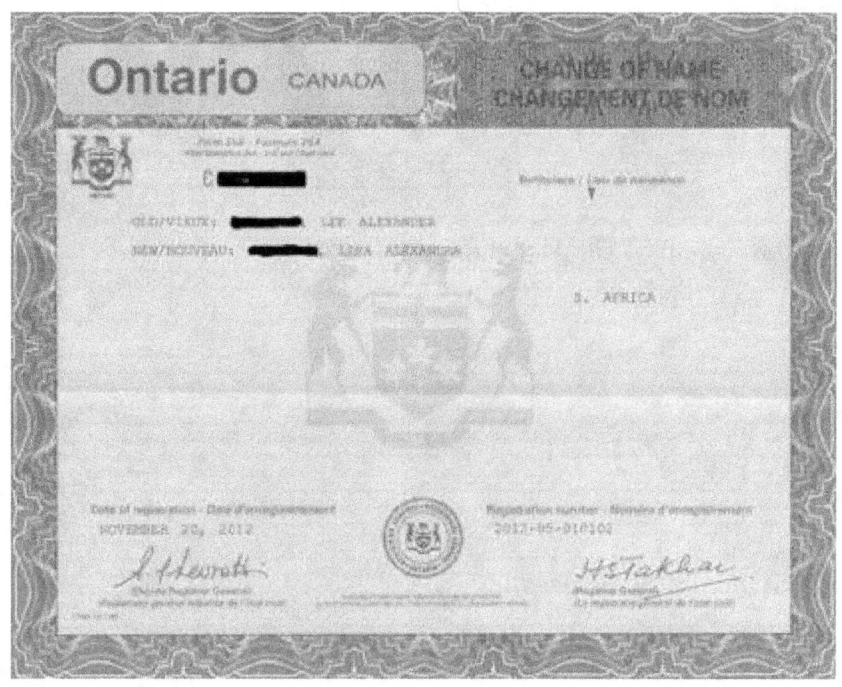

Figure 9 Legal Name Change Certificate

There it was my new name, Lisa Alexandra!

These were tears of sorrow and joy. Sorrow filled my heart, knowing well that this meant the end of Lee Alexander's life. Joy for the birth of Lisa Alexandra a woman. This was an extremely emotional time for me. Other transgender women explained to me that they also went through a stage of mourning. They mourned the death of their previous lives. Leah would later explain to me months later, that she actually mourned the end of Lee; a friend she missed dearly. As time had passed, she grew to accept and love me as Lisa in the same way she had with Lee. I immediately picked up my phone and texted

Leah and Nancy. My phone beeped with the immediate response from Leah:

Me
I am now legally Lisa Alexandra

Leah
Really

Me
I sent a picture of the certificate

Leah
WOw

Leah
Wow

Me
I am crying tears of joy. A very emotional time

Leah
Hahaha, that's cause you are a woman fool. That's what girls do

Next, I had to call Tammy and tell her the news, my voice still filled with emotion. She was so happy to hear my good news.

"Now I have to call you Lisa, no more Lee." I could hear the happiness in her voice. "Thank you for sharing this special moment with me." She continued to say.

Next was to scan the document and inform my Therapist Sandy. Now I needed to send this document along with the testimonials I had received from my electrolysist at Niagara Skin Institute that does my laser hair removal. Just the past Friday Sandy had sent me a copy of her testimonial that she was sending to CAMH. It read:

"TO WHOM IT MAY CONCERN:
RE: LISA ALEXANDRA DOB March 6, 1962

Lisa Alexandra has been a client of mine since July 17, 2012. During our first session, she advised me that she was in the process of transitioning to the female gender. She presented in female attire, makeup, and wig. She told me that she is receiving electrolysis treatments and makeup and wardrobe advice to assist in her transition.

Ms. Alexandra has since attended at my office on a regular basis, to discuss this process and her awareness of the issues surrounding it. She is obviously very comfortable with her decision and taking correct steps to ensure that her new life will be comfortable for those in her life as well.

Ms. Alexandra is a high functioning, well spoken, introspective individual, who has thoughtfully made this life changing decision to become congruent in herself - identity. She states that she is well supported by family, friends and a network of professionals.

Ms. Alexandra's decision to transition has come at a point in her life where she has the maturity, life experience, and self-awareness to do what is right for her. As her therapist, I fully support her as she moves forward in this direction. Should you require additional information in this regard, please do not hesitate to contact me.

Sincerely,"

27 November 2012, Tuesday

Legally me: The certificate gave me a new found confidence as Lisa. I went to check on my first healthy vending machine I had placed. I then proceeded to visit two other businesses, dropping off brochures for the Healthy vending machines. I had become a confidant woman. Nothing would hold this woman back.

2-9 December 2012

Final trip to Curacao: I was fortunate to have two friends who accompanied me on my final trip, T&T. Tammy and Tatiana who were awesome friends that supported me in my decision to proceed on my new journey. The trip went off well ending the week with a Farewell barbecue as I successfully spun the story to these friends that I will soon be heading up north to live with the Indians. I was surprised at how well I was able to spin the story with conviction and believe. Even Tammy commented that she was even beginning to believe my story. I explained to her that it was not a total lie as Vee had invited me to visit her family up north, who are part Native American decent. Lee is going away, and the lady that will be looking after my condo and business is no other than Lisa.

I asked my friends to give me their physical mailing address as I will not be available through any electronic means. Resorting back to communication methods we used to use just over twenty years ago. Sending postcards or letters, even though it could take as long as three weeks before the other party received it, add another three weeks to receive a reply. It was a very interesting concept my friends embraced. Most of them were really intrigued by the idea that I will be away from modern civilization for so long. Many of them wishing they could join me on this new adventure.
Now with the trip over, there is no reason to switch back to Lee. The day after I arrived back I was comfortably back in the role of Lisa.

11 December 2012 Tuesday
Services Ontario: This was the day I would go change my license, health card and car registration to Lisa. On 30 November my Doctor gave me the letter that I needed for the Ministry of Transport along with my name change certificate. I picked up ticket number 27, one

of my lucky numbers. Would this be my lucky day? I arrived with number 8 showing, so I had a long wait ahead. I had the gut feeling that the hand written letter from my Doctor would not be sufficient. This proved to be the case as it did not mention my new gender to be "female" only that I was transgendering. Margret who attended to me was very helpful from Services Ontario. She told me that when I return on Friday with the correct letter, she will attend to me immediately, as she would be working at the dealer's registration desk.

Back home I searched up on the Internet to make sure I get the letter done right this time. I emailed the following information to my Doctor requesting a new letter.

*If you are undergoing or have completed sex reassignment surgery, and want to change the sex designation on your driver's license, bring the following documents to a **Service Ontario center**:*

• A letter from you specifying the change requested. This letter needs to include your full name, current address, driver's license number and the name and address of the physician who has signed an opinion letter in support of the change.

• A letter, on the letterhead of a physician licensed by the College of Physicians and Surgeons of Ontario, and signed by the physician, in which the physician states that:

--the physician has examined or treated the driver who is requesting the change in sex designation on the driver's license, and

--it is the opinion of the physician that the change in the sex designation on the driver's license is appropriate.

Your application will be reviewed to ensure that the documents meet requirements.

Full surgery is not required as a condition for sex designation changes.

13 December 2012 Thursday

Correct letter: At 12pm I picked up the new letter from my Doctor's Niagara Falls office. It read:

ATTN: Ministry of transportation

This letter is in regards to the sex designation change for Lisa Alexandra (formally Lee Alexandra) on her Ontario Driver's License.

I, Dr. M B, have examined and treated the driver, Lisa (Lee) Alexandra, who is requesting the change in sex designation from male to female on her Ontario Driver's License. It is my opinion that the change of sex designation to female on the Ontario Driver's License is appropriate for Lisa Alexandra.

Sincerely

(signed Dr. B)

14 December 2012 Friday

A good day: I arrived at Services Ontario confident and ready for the change. Margret recognized me immediately and invited me to sit down. All went smoothly, having to take two new photos of me for my license and heath card. I had to sign the new documents commenting, the only changes were my first, middle and gender. I jokingly commented to her, "It is a pity my birth date won't change!" "Don't we all wish to be younger," was her cheerful reply

I left her desk a happy woman; my temporary Driver's License had the Lisa and sex "F". In a few days or weeks, I would receive the new documents.

17- 21 Dec 2012

Name changes: I had an excel list that I had used to check off my address change when I moved to the Falls. So I added a Lisa column for my name changes. This week I managed to change my name on my Social Insurance Number (SIN), American Express, insurances, mobile phone, Hertz Gold card and my Author account with Author House for the first book I published. I informed my book consultant about my transgender change. He saw this as a positive to use to promote my book and this one that I am working on.

On the 19th I finally received a reply from the Netherlands Consulate with regards to changing my passport. It looks like it is more complicated than what I thought, knowing that the Dutch are normally quite liberal and tolerable nation. I have to petition the Dutch courts to requests my gender change for my passport. Well, it might be complicated, but it is something I have to do.

21 December 2012, Thursday
Christmas Show: I managed to get tickets for Tammy and me for the Christmas Dinner Show at Oh Canada on Lundy's Lane. The only seats available were the prime seats right in front at the horseshoe tables. This was the first time that Tammy and I went out together as two women. I wore my red top, black skirt with the fleece pantyhose. This was a good chance for me to wear my new winter boots I had recently bought. A sexy black pair, wedge knee height, with fur lining on the top. They had a wedge heel that made me feel sexy when walking in them; they had the ideal sole for the ice. I have to say even though I am tall, I love to wear heels, even just a 3" as it makes you feel sexy and give me the feminine confidence I need.

We called a taxi as I wanted to enjoy myself and have a few drinks to get into the Christmas spirit. A pretty female driver picked us up. She explained that her father who is the dispatcher only assigns female passengers for her. Wow, I thought I must have pulled off my female voice quite well when I called in for the cab.

My only worry was that with the seats right in the front, I hoped that I would not be pulled up on stage for audience participation. The show and food were great, served up as you would have a family dinner, dishing up yourself, passing the various dishes around the table that we shared with another family. During the intermission, I went to the bathroom for a pee. I could hear the woman in the stall next to me. I soon learned that a woman's flow can be as strong as a male's. For some crazy reason, I always presumed women would have a weaker flow.

"You really look great as a beautiful woman. I can see you are happy as Lisa, as I can see the twinkle in your eyes." was the comforting comment I received from, Tammy. The show really put us into the Christmas spirit and what made it even better was when we stepped out of the show. We were greeted by the white of all the snow on the ground. What a beautiful sight with all the night lights, it has snowed while we were in the show. Another female driver picked us up to take us back home. A perfect ending to a great night.

21 December 2012, Friday
Christmas cards: I had to go out and buy a few Christmas cards as I had received 4 cards addressed to Lee from neighbors on the same floor as me. The decision was made; I dropped off 4 Christmas cards

for the neighbors under their doors, signed by Lisa. This had a payoff as I bumped into one of my neighbors the next day while doing my laundry. I did not bother to put on the hairpiece or makeup. I was greeted as Lisa. The neograft hair transplant had taken root, and the hair in the front was growing. So even without the top hair piece I had a female look to my hair. Soon the Lee look will no longer exist.

24-26 December 2012

Christmas: Even though my son was sick we managed to spend quality family time together over Christmas and Boxing Day. Just hanging out at home and watching movies. Christmas night we decided to go out and watch the movie everyone was raving about, "The Hobbit." We both enjoyed it and even though it is almost three hours long, the movie was able to keep you captivated to the full, leaving you hanging at the end.

27 December 2012 Friday

Confrontation: I receive at the text from my son while I was doing my vending as Lisa. He asked me if I could take him to the walk-in clinic. It was just a few days earlier he had finally broken his silence on my transgender change. When he told me, he does not want to see me as Lisa as it would freak him out. Being to optimist that I am I looked at the positive side to this. He is finally talking about my changes. This is how the conversation went:

Bret

Can you take me to the walk-in clinic? I might have acute bronchitis

Me

Yes, I can, but I am doing my vending so I am your aunt at the moment.

Bret

Then forget about it

Me

ok sorry. I can change later and take you.

Bret

No, I just rather not see you; I have too much pain of what you just told me now. I have no more mother or father neither a family to rely on, so I hope you understand now why I'm so depressed.

Me

I do understand, and it pains me. I have been dealing with this internal turmoil all my life. I can change and come for you now.

Bret

No, leave it and forget about it I'll walk.

Me

At least take a taxi I will pay you back later.

That conversation left me questioning what I was doing. I debated the decision I had made through my mind. I methodically was going over the two options: 1. to proceed with my gender change knowing very well I am truly happy, but at the cost of my son's happiness. 2. I halt the change and revert back to being Lee just for the sake of my son, knowing well I would have to live the rest of my life dealing with the internal turmoil. "No I must stay on my path; I knew from the start that this road will not be easy. There will be plenty of obstacles or negativities I will have to overcome. Bret will eventually come around and accept me for who I am" was my final thoughts. I have come a long way for me to turn back now. Why should I go back and serve my life sentence in the wrong gender? The time was approaching when I would have to have a heart to heart talk with Bret and tell him my true feelings.

30 December 2012, Sunday

The time is right. I was so happy when my son accepted my invitation to have a late breakfast together. 1pm was the set time; this was my opportunity to take advantage of him breaking his silence and tell him how I feel before he could shut down again.

We decided on our regular Diner"The Early Bird" that serves a great steak and eggs. I thought about trying something different today but decided on going for the regular knowing that I will enjoy it. As usual, we started off with coffee. I did not have to look at the menu to order mine: steak medium, eggs over easy, brown toast with the side order of onions and mushroom. The steak & eggs also came with fried potatoes. I am not a big fan of hash browns, but their fried potatoes are tasty, a bit of salt and ketchup always adds to the flavor. Bret ordered the same with the exception of whole wheat toast.

He began to tell me of his ambition to make a media empire in the next twenty years. I was happy to hear that he said my situation drove him to work towards his independence and become successful.

"Our family history destined me for greatness. Like our great-great grandfather Alexander Thompson who was awarded the Victoria Cross" Alexander Thompson was awarded the VC during the Indian Mutiny as quoted from Wikipedia:

Thompson was about 34 years old, and a <u>lance-corporal</u> in the <u>42nd Regiment of Foot</u> (later The <u>Black Watch</u> (Royal Highlanders)), <u>British Army</u> during the <u>Indian Mutiny</u> when the following deed took place for which he was awarded the VC. On 15 April 1858 during the attack on <u>Fort Ruhya</u>, <u>British India</u>, Lance-Corporal Thompson volunteered, with others, including <u>Edward Spence</u>, to assist Captain <u>William Martin Cafe</u> in carrying in the body of a lieutenant from the

top of the <u>glacis</u>, in an exposed position under heavy fire. His
citation read:

For daring gallantry, on the 10th April, 1858, when at the attack of
the Fort of Ruhya, in having volunteered to assist Captain Groves,
Commanding the 4th Punjab Rifles, in bringing in the body of
Lieutenant Willoughby, of that Corps, from the top of the Glacis, in a
most exposed situation, under a heavy fire.

He was also proud of his grandpa's intelligence, being able to create
electronic devices and my Uncle Jimmy who was a very successful
businessman. Both my son and I had Alexander as our middle
names. All I could do is look at him with pride and admiration,
knowing that I being an optimist was rubbing off on him.
I was able to explain to him that nobody can understand the internal
struggle I have had to endure for all these years. The change is
making me truly happy. Before my decision to move ahead with the
change, my life was not going anywhere. He told me that he will try
and not let this bother him; he has to move on with his own life. I
also explained to him that like him when I first arrived in Curacao I
had no family. I created my own family as he will be able to do the
same. My only recommendation was for him to have more kids. Not
like me just having one son.
"This is how I look like when I am the other person." referring to my
natural look without my top hair piece or makeup. Slowly my face

was starting to be more feminine even to the point that when I look into the mirror when I have to be Lee for him. In the reflection, I am starting to see Lisa shining through. It was just two days ago when I entered a store that knew me as Lee. The female store owner and I would previously have a friendly conversation. So when I entered as Lisa, she did not seem startled or even notice the change. We had our regular idle chit chat as before.

I made the promise that when we meet up, I will come to him as Lee. Knowing well that all I needed to do was just not dress feminine or wear makeup. But there will come a day when I cannot hide my breasts that I have started to notice the growth. Predicting that in two more months they will become more noticeable. At that point, I am hoping he will finally accept me for who I really am.

31 December, Tuesday
New Year: I had a quiet New Year's Eve with just Nancy and Pauline. I had something to show off to my two girlfriends. With the help of my black padded bra, I had tits. The pain and sensitivity I was experiencing behind my nipples had gone away. My breasts still small but with the padded bra they gave me an A-B size. I had to let them feel my growing breast. Nancy wanted to see them in the flesh which I was so happy to show her. She felt them and commented on how firm they were.

We were able to see all the fireworks from my patio bringing in the New Year. Nancy had predicted, "Next new year the three of us will have partners for the next few years."

Later that night she said, "If we don't have anyone then you and I will have to end up together."

"But you will have to accept me without my penis." I replied

"Yeah but you will have better tits than me, " she looked over at me with her cute naughty smile

1 January 2013, Tuesday

Good food. Vee invited me to her place yesterday as she had friends over from work .She had plenty of food to eat. Three of her coworkers were chefs so the food was excellent. We had crab legs, prime rib, coconut shrimp, bacon wrapped scallops, mash potatoes (my favorite) and meatballs that one of Vee's girlfriends had made with her secret recipe source. There were so many crab legs that I was able to take some home. Now I could say that Vee gave me crabs.

2 January 2012, Wednesday

A smile to my face: There was just one white envelope in the mailbox and one junk mail flier which went straight into the bin located at the mailbox. I could feel through the envelope that there was a card inside. I did not know which card it was as the envelope was just had the PO Box return address from Kingston, Ontario. This must be my Health Card I thought, but when I opened it I immediately recognized the Ontario Driver' license. My first official ID as Lisa and most important of all listing my gender as "F". This just brought a big smile to my face.

Chapter Seven

A New Year A New Life

2013 a New Year a new life Will this be the year that I finally reach the goal of becoming a complete woman? Switching gender has some interesting adjustments one has to make when switching from male to female. Here is a list of some of them:

- **Handbags.** Having to carry a handbag for your wallet/purse, keys, etc.. Gone are the days of just putting your wallet and keys in your pockets. With most women clothing I have noticed they don't have pockets. Now I have to get used to carrying a bag around me, or if I am just going over to the supermarket or shop, I will have my purse in hand. I now have to worry about losing my bag, purse keys and all.

- **Peeing sitting down.** It might sound easy, but I when I would sit down to pee, my brain was telling me I needed to shit. It had taken a while before my brain and bladder were in sync just to pee.

- **Ladies first.** In my previous gender role I was normally a courteous person, stepping aside for woman or allowing a person to go before me. The old saying "ladies first". Now I have gentleman holding doors for me allowing me to right of way.

• **Hit on.** This one I just had to accept, even though I am only attracted to women. I mostly have older men chatting me up. So I decided to take these gestures or comments as a compliment. When I was entering Casino Niagara in the summer wearing my 4' heels. I overheard the comment from a gentleman in a group, "I could tap that". All I could do is smile and laugh internally.

The process to change my Dutch passport to reflect my new name and gender proved to be more complex than I thought. The frustrating part was that my lawyer would base my petition on the Dutch law requirements, whereas in Canada the transgender process is different. I was almost about to give up and accept the fact the fact that I cannot leave the country until I have my Canadian citizenship. In January I finally sent my new application with my new name and gender. I now had the adequate time in Canada needed to apply; this is about three years on the last four years.

One of the requirements was that I needed to have a letter from a GID expert that is registered in the Netherlands. When my lawyer received my email showing my frustration. I told him there is no way I will revert back to male just to travel to the Netherlands so that an expert can assess me and give the opinion needed for the courts.

She contacted the courts on the complex international situation I was in. Fortunately, the petition came back with a positive response that they will accept the letters from my Doctor and therapist. All these complex issues resulted in extra lawyer fees. I often wonder if it is just the lawyers that make things more complex than what they really are, just to collect extra fees from the client. After I stated to her that I was not a wealthy person and that I had plenty of expenses dealing with my transition. Every time I would request a letter from my doctor, she would charge me $25 for a letter, eventually charging me $100 for a letter when she had to show that she is a member of the College of Physicians of Ontario .Surprising to me and associates in the vending business, my new business venture was growing fast.

My friend Harry commented, "Is it because you are a woman?"
I think it has to do with my positive attitude and my new fearless attitude. As Lee, I always felt that I had the potential to do well in business, but I felt that something was always holding me back. I would wonder if it was fear, fear of doing well? Like a thoroughbred racehorse, I felt the will and power to run as fast as possible, but the unviable jockey was holding the reigns. Now I am free as Lisa no reigns to hold me back, I can sprint ahead free.

For a person who cannot understand my new found freedom I could explain it in this way. My previous life as a male was like a prisoner serving a life sentence, knowing very well freedom was not in sight.

How does a prisoner deal with mentally knowing they can never be free? They accept their situation and make the best of a bad situation "adapt or die." Caged in my male body I had accepted what I was dealt with, a woman caged in this body never to be free. In some ways, you could describe it as a form of Stockholm syndrome. For forty-five years I had made the best of my situation, living a happy, productive light.

Then in July 2012 my prison door swung free, freedom had come. Finally, after years of serving my life sentence as a male, I can now live free as a female.

Caged no more
I have no door
I am finally free
So let it be
Free as bird
My tattoo says the word
FREE!

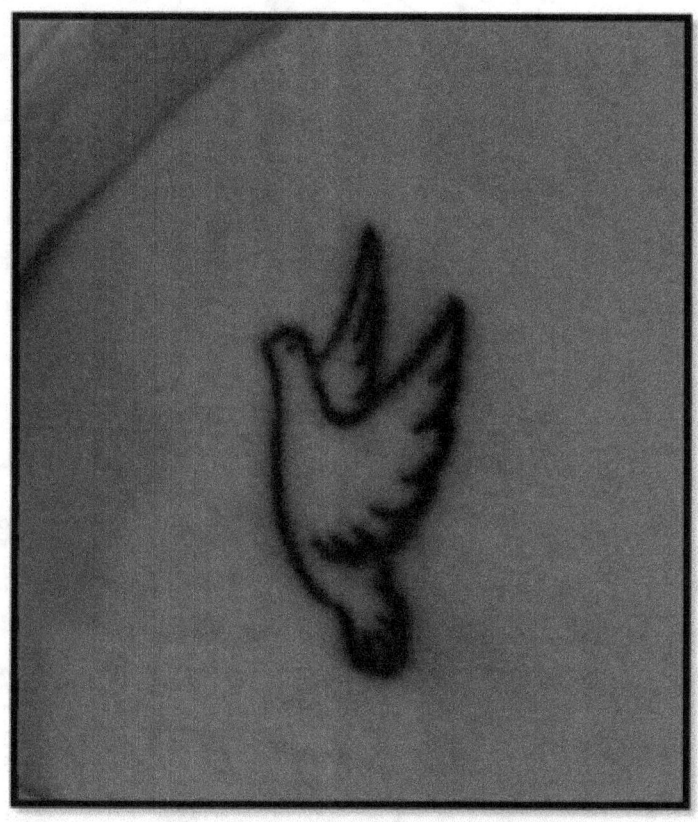

Figure 10 Tattoo January 2013

The dreaded day 27th of March 2012 rolled in. This was the day I had to appear in court for the accident charged with failing to yield which if convicted could carry a maximum fine of $5000. Surprisingly I felt good that morning. I had planned not to work that morning even though my court time was 2:30pm. I felt the confidence knowing that I was not in the wrong. It was Lee that had the accident, but Lisa was the one to stand trial.

I met my paralegal in the waiting room, a pleasant gentleman from Road Warriors. We briefly discussed my case, noting that I had to be firm on the idea that I did not leave the road when turning into the parking lot. The construction cone was the one that should be on trial I thought. It was the one that made me stop, causing me to reverse a bit thus causing the collision. Ted went into the courtroom to speak to the Prosecutor to see if the witness were present. Surprisingly he came back with a proposal from the Prosecutor. She was prepared to drop the charge to the equivalency of a parking ticket. No deterrent points lost on my license. I jumped at the opportunity to just get the day over and the dark cloud above my head to fade away.

I entered the court with Ted waiting for my case to proceed. The proposed deal was presented to the Judge who had agreed on it. But he asked if Lee was present, only then did Ted inform the Judge that I now went by the name Lisa. I stood a confident woman before the Judge stating my name "Lisa." After I had entered my plea of guilty, the fine was presented to me. I did not waste time paying the fine immediately at the courthouse and left a relieved woman. The road ahead was now paved smooth, my journey back on track.

The next week I drove up to Toronto with my friend Tammy to see Gerald Isaac, a vocal coach highly recommended by my Therapist Sandy and her daughter. There we met Gerald and his wife Shea a sweet couple that you could see was a match made in heaven. Tammy sat in with me during our discussion; positive energy was filled in the small 10' x 30' studio located in a quiet suburb of Toronto. There was such a good chemistry between us. Even though I had a reply from a clinic that specialized in voice lessons for transgender patients. I knew right then that this beautiful couple will be the ones to help me find my true Lisa voice.

A new woman had entered my life; an aunt of Nancy from Halifax was visiting. Nancy knew right off the bat that Dee and I would hit it off together. She was in her late forties, divorced with grown up kids. To top it off she was a sister friend a term I would soon learn that explains a lesbian. Nancy and I had picked her up at the Toronto Pearson airport in my van. Nancy had not told Dee that I was a transgender woman. She confessed to me soon after we got to know each other that she was now aware I was a trans woman when we first met. It was only when I bent down to get a beer out of Nancy's fridge that she noticed something a bit manly. I had stopped wearing my hip pads due to the discomfort. The upper wide torso at the time had given away my secret.

She accompanied me to what would turn out to be my first and only voice lesson with Gerald. I just could not afford the monthly expense of driving up every week for an hour lesson or every two weeks for a two-hour session. I just could not afford the time either as I was hard at work trying to establish my new business. Needless to say, the lesson was very interesting and productive. I soon came to realize what an actor or actress must go through to perfect the speech for rolls. It was interesting to learn that there is a simple exercise of saying "hello" in so many ways:

- Do I know you?
- I haven't seen you in ages
- Thank god I haven't seen you in ages
- I can't believe that you didn't get that joke

Over the three weeks, Dee and I forged a new friendship with both of us learning from each other. She would learn to understand more about transgender woman. Early in our friendship days on the trip to Toronto for my first voice lesson, she made a comment to me that was a bit hurtful. "It will not be a lesbian that you will end up but an open minded woman, as a lesbian would not go for a man dressed as a woman." But she would soon learn to understand us transgender woman that we are not just a "man dressed as a woman" but to our minds, we are "women." It is just that our bodies that we were born with did not match up to our minds. About two weeks later she would make a comment to after she got to know more about me.

"You are such a girl" she commented after I told her I had minor cosmetic surgery to remove an unsightly small lump from my left leg. This comment was not only just music to my ears, but reassured me that her opinion of me as a transgender woman had changed. She was now seeing me as a woman.

In return, I learn a bit about the lesbian lifestyle and the most important lesson of all! How do I fend off a male trying to chat me up? I was sitting in TJ's during karaoke night when I was approached by a man, "I like your boobies, I want to suck your boobies." A funny thought I had later was that I could have pulled out one of my breast forms and said, "Suck on this baby." Dee soon came to my rescue while I just sat back as I watched how she handles his advances on her. The simple and diplomatic way, was to ease the tension from an advance was to say to the man is "Hey man I am like you I like girls too."

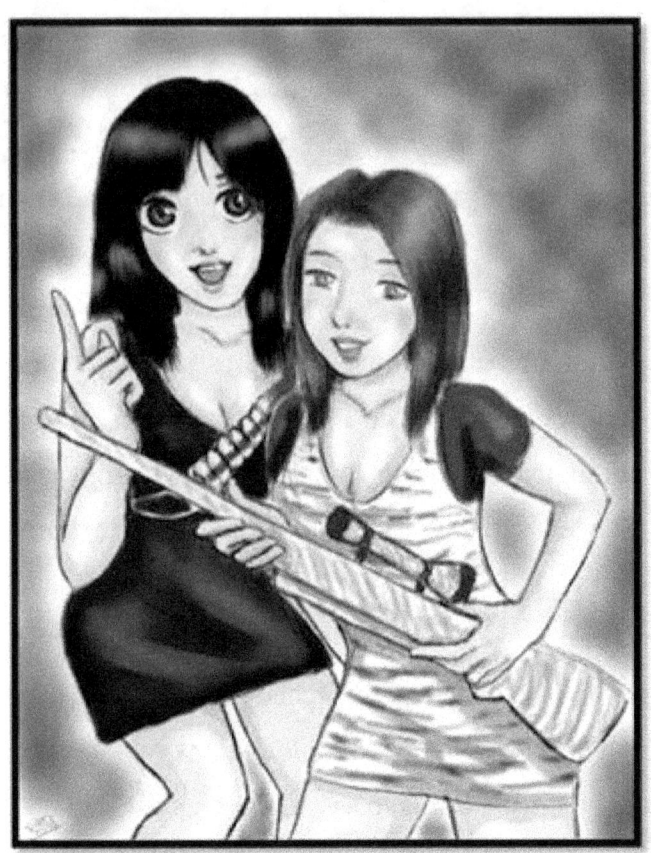

Figure 11 Lisa & Dee

10 May 2013, Friday

Adult party Attended another party at Mistress Avaya and Master Blaze's house. Not knowing what to expect turned out to be a new beautiful awakening for me. I met another transgender woman Alison. Alison was two years into hormone treatment, she had noticeable breast development. The party moved down to the basement dungeon. There I had my true intermit time with a beautiful dark haired woman Tammy. What a beautiful experience.

16 May 2013, Thursday

Boob trip. Over a week ago I had posted on FB

Lisa Alexandra

May 8 at 8:51pm •

To get bigger boobs or not to?

That is the question.

Leah TO GET !!!!!!

May 8 at 9:10pm

Nigel 36d ?

May 8 at 11:48pm

Di What question? Lee just do it!

May 9 at 12:41am

Dee Lisa, always, always do what feels right to you!!!

May 9 at 7:50am

Lisa Alexandra Thanks for the support, good news is that my boob credit was approved, so I am off to Toronto next Wednesday to see the surgeon. They will let me try on different sizes to see what shape and size I want. Probably going for the new gummy bear implants as they say they feel so natural.

May 9 at 9:25am • Like

Dee That's awesome Lisa, you should book a voice lesson while you're going to be there.

May 9 at 11:00am •

Lisa Alexandra Dee, I am doing just that. I am doing my voice lesson first, and then off to see the surgeon.

May 9 at 1:37pm

Tammy Looking very forward to accompany you on your next big adventure!!

May 9 at 2:30pm

Miss T Hey congrats how do I get a boob credit?

Monday at 10:33pm

Lisa Alexandra Maybe OLG could start a Boob Lottery

Monday at 11:40pm

The internal debate had begun. All the positive comments that followed my post validated my decision I knew I was about to make. Alison's two-year development justified my research results. It would take about two years before I would reach my peak in breast development. With this expectation in mind, it was not the size I wanted. I wanted them bigger, summer was upon us. I so wanted to flaunt my new breast, having the freedom to wear the dresses and tops I only fantasized about wearing. The decision was made, and I had to go to Toronto to see Dr. Martin Jugenburg at Toronto Cosmetic Surgery Institute. I had vigorously researched who was the best surgeon in Toronto to see. My trip back in August 2012 had confirmed my decision. They were located in the Fairmont York Hotel, a very well professional, clean and modern establishment; staffs were friendly and helpful and to top it off you did not have to pay for a consultation. A true testament that they are confident in their results.

Tammy accompanied me on the trip to see Kim. It was a surgery day so the Doctor was busy. The main goal is to try on different sizes of implants. Tammy had also commented on how clean and organized their establishment was. It was decided beforehand that I would not go for the saline implants recommended for the male body. I wanted the silicone implants referred to as "gummy bears". Due to their jelly like feel, giving you the natural breast feel.

After some measurements and testing, it was determined the 650cc was the best option for me. This would give me a size D breast. Due to my upper body size, it was not recommended to go too small, nor did I want to go too big. D was perfect for me. I left the office a happy content woman. I had to move forward. The next day I would see my Dr. I needed to discuss with her about my possible future breast development over the next year or so.

The very next day I went to see Dr. B and explained to her my wish to proceed with my breasts. My main concern was; was it too early to do them now knowing that they are still developing. I asked her if I could show her my breasts, which she did consent. She was very happy with my development. But felt it was too early to do it and suggested I wait another seven months. Which at that point would mark the second anniversary when I officially started taking hormones. Seven months would be December, a perfect month as this would be the slowest time for my vending business. It would take about six weeks to fully recuperate as you cannot lift anything heavy during that time. I informed Kim at the Cosmetic Surgery who concurred that I must respect my Doctors decision as she has my best interest at heart. She went on to say "Time flies. December will be here before you know."

Other negatives would become positive: Just two days before my friend Helen had done me the favor of informing my friends, a couple that lived in Curacao, I had known for over twenty-five years, that I was transgender. I had dreaded telling them as my gut instinct knew they would not take it well and that I would be subject to them making fun at my expense. Fortunate my friend Vee who had become my transgender mentor was sleeping over. She was there to console me when I received the Skype message from here informing it went as expected. It created tension that night after she had told them over drinks at the scenic bar at the Rif Fort that overlooks the Curaçao harbor entrance. The woman had reacted in a burst of laughter while the man was quick to inform the waitress "Oh my God my friend wants to get his cock cut off!"

Vee comforted me that I should not let them put me down, it was expected that there will be people who would react in a negative or humiliating way towards me. I could not hold back my emotions I was so angry at their reactions even though it was expected. The anger gave way to tears as Vee reached out to hold my hand to comfort me. "Why are people so cruel?" I thought. Many thoughts raced through my mind, how I should respond to this negativity. Should I just leave it be as suggested by Vee or should I make my thoughts know to them? In no time the words came to me. I logged onto my old Facebook account to message Valerie. I posted the following

"Hi Valerie out of respect for Bret PLEASE do not broadcast to the world what Helen told you. It is very personal what I am dealing with for the past 45 years. One by one I have been contacting all my friends. Today I tried to reach you and Sam. All other 28 friends have responded in a very respectable and supporting way. I don't expect you to understand or accept this difficult decision I had to

151

make in my life. Once again please respect Bret's privacy. We as a family are dealing with it in our own loving way. I am very happy in my new life, finally free from my life imprisonment I had to endure for the last 45 years."

It was one of my regular moments we shared over lunch which had become special to me. I would not pressure him on my changes but instead take the time to cherish the moment as a parent. We both enjoyed the roast lamb special at a Greek restaurant we would occasionally visit. At the end of the meal I used the male restroom as I was "dressed down". I would wear my not so feminine female jeans, black t-shirt, white sneakers and a hoodie to hide my ever growing boobs. The only makeup was my concealer and a bit of powder to smooth over complexion. While I washed my hands, I looked into the mirror. The reflection revealed more of Lisa; the image of Lee was fading away. Soon there would be no way to even try and look like Lee.

On the drive back from the restaurant I finally had the opportunity to clarify what I had said to Bret the previous lunch meeting when I said to him. "You have to understand that it is getting more difficult for me to try and return back to me for you when we meet." He had responded that he did not understand what I meant. At that moment I decided just to leave it and not try to explain it to him. The seed was planted for our next conversation. Now this day was my chance to clarify to him, "what I meant the last time was that you know there are physical changes happening to me?"

He acknowledged it with a simple "yes", one word that would carry a lot of weight. I was immediately overwhelmed with joy sensing that he was slowly starting to accept my transformation. I would see him again as soon as three days' time when I would give him a lift to college.

On my return home I was greeted by an email from Sam using my Lisa email address he must have received from Helen. Tears of joy filled my eyes as the positive emotion rippled through my body. He and Valerie would respect my wished; they were shocked by the news of my life change. I must just give them time to absorb the news and to come to terms with it. I just had to share my joy with my dear friend Tammy who has been with me all the way through my transition so far. I picked up the phone; I struggled to speak to her the emotions over joy drowning out my ability to speak.

I do have to acknowledge that every person that I personally told had an easier time coming to terms with this. It was now time for me to reach out to my brother. We have never been the closest of siblings. My sister Elizabeth was the one to inform him at a coffee shop after they had both finished work. He was absolutely shocked, to the point that Elizabeth was worried that he was going to have heart attack. It was the constant shock theme that everyone was going through after they were informed. Nobody had any clue what I was going through all the past forty-five years. I sent him the message through my old Skype profile telling that I would like to speak to him if he was up to it.

I pulled into the parking lot of my hairdresser for my weekly appointment if I had the funds for the wash and dry. For the past four years, I have been going to the hair salon that is run by a few Latin American women. I always have a love and soft spot for a Latin American woman. While I was reversing into the parking, I was unaware that Gia and Gabriella were watching when they made the comment and acknowledgment. "The hormones must be working she parks like a woman."

To be honest, I am so bad at reverse parking, and when I see that I have not parked well, I did comment to my friend Tammy one day while parking by the beer store. The car was parked slightly askew. "I don't have to park perfectly I am now a woman. I did my driver's license test at the age of 18. I was lucky that the examining officer who did my road test first and ended off with a reverse parking. I did the test in my small blue mini. When I finally completed the reverse parking, the oversized officer turned to me and said, "You are the worst person I had for parking" To my surprise, he actually still passed me. From then on when I needed to park I would jump out of the driver's seat and let my friend Grant Park for me. Sorry ladies I just had to mention about the parking.

154

Hormones were having another effect on me, I was becoming more emotional. In the past, I would get a lump in my throat when watching a particular movie scene. Hell, now I cry like a girl, even when I become emotional about anything I can easily resort to tears. New people are entering into my life, my circle of friends forever expanding. In ten months as Lisa, I had met or made friends with more people than the five years as Lee since I moved to Canada. There is Alison, another transgender woman who actually started hormones the very same month as me in December 2011. But in my case, I had the two-month break in between. So I would consider her to be two months ahead of me. We had met at a party and soon formed a special friendship as we realized we have so much in common. We both had lived heterosexual lives in the past with strong male sex drives. We were both able to share our experiences with each other or support each other when times are tough.

A few weeks later I met a gay couple Dave & Jeremy who I would refer to as my DJs. This was a triangle friendship that we felt was destiny. Jeremy and I connected in so many ways as we shared some similarities in the past. Like me he had lived the heterosexual life and had lost a daughter at the young age of nineteen, I had lost my niece when she was just nineteen. Dave would become my gay best friend that most women want. He would advise me on my looks and what to wear and would always compliment me on my beauty.

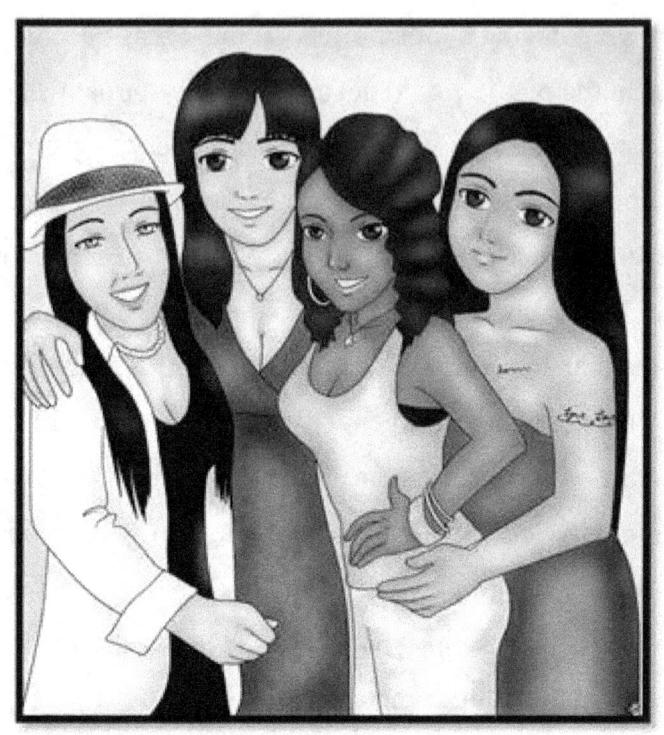

Figure 12 Girls Night Out Dee, Lisa, Tara & Nancy

Chapter Eight

Woman Inside Takes Over

Sixteen months on hormones I feel more beautiful as changes take effect. Food was starting to taste even better, with certain flavors exploding in my mouth. I was with Tammy at the Mandarin Buffet when I sliced off a piece of the prime rib and placed into my mouth. The taste exploded into my mouth, I looked up to Tammy and said, "I just experience a taste orgasm." I discussed this with a friend Bella I had met online through the Charlie Spice online radio show. Bella is a pro-Dominatrix, who does most of her BDSM session online through Skype and has her Twitter account @BigBellaNova. We were both co-host on the show. The show was all about the sex and the sex industry. As an author of "Putas of the Caribbean" I had the knowledge and experiences needed for the show. Bella and I immediately stuck up a friendship calling each other regularly through Skype video calls. It did not take us long to start the "BellaLisa Show" titled The BellaLisaShow. Interestingly Bella had experienced taste orgasms but unlike mine. She actually became extremely moist between the legs. Hers occurred while she was having dinner with a friend at a restaurant while dining on seafood. I discovered red wine has a more appealing taste to me now. I now see why so many females I know enjoy the occasional glass of red wine.

Along the road, I have met a few more women that have claimed to have experienced taste orgasms.

I had to take my breasts, waist and hip measurements for my Doctor for my quarterly checkup which coincides with my regular blood tests. I was thrilled to see that I had increased by an inch on my hips and breasts. My waist had decreased by an inch. Looking at the mirror, I can see the hourglass starting to take shape. This only adds to my feeling of being a woman both body and soul.

My sex drive returned but this time, my brain is now rewired in a more fem way. My attraction for females is as strong as ever, reassuring me that I am a lesbian. I kept an open mind as it is known that some transgender do experience sexual preference switch. But now instead of having an erection, I feel an internal sensation within the head of my penis. Alison who is a few months ahead of me on hormones had told me she was started experiencing becoming wet like a woman, I now have the same. Feeling so feminine and sexy one night. I experience what I call my first female orgasm through masturbation, with the help on my Conair massager. Unlike a male orgasm that explodes in a quick rush sensation as you ejaculate. My orgasm lingered on for about ten times longer than a male's orgasm. Unable to ejaculate now I experience the orgasm body and mind.

Sandy, my therapist, had sparked a new interest in me. She had toyed with the idea that we should do a TV show that she could produce titled "This is Lisa". Well, enthusiasm took over; I just had to try it out. I hooked up with my friend Alison and did a YouTube test show titled "The Lisa & Alison Show". I did an interview with Alison about her transgender change. I had prepared the questions and emailed them to her. We just had one test run of the questions over the phone. We met at my place and with no rehearsal video recorded our first show. The show lasted about 21 minutes.

Dave and Jeremy joined us for the second show, which we did as a spur of the moment. We had started having an interesting conversation about gay relationships compared to heterosexual relationships. I quickly paused the conversation as I said that this would make a perfect show discussion on how straight couples could learn from gay couples. In no time I had my Canon camera on the tripod and filming began. Then we realized the camera was not recording, so we had to repeat all that we had discussed in the first few minutes. Surprisingly this unscripted conversation which naturally took on a similar format as "The View" last about 20 minutes. I immediately noticed that Dave, Jeremy and I had chemistry on camera. We had no problem picking up on a totally unscripted conversation. Alison still seemed a bit more reserved, not jumping in on the conversations.

Saturday 6 July which also my sixth anniversary the day I became a landed immigrant in Canada. My DJs and I drove up to Toronto. The plan was to stay in a motel near Woodbine Racetrack for the night before the Queen's Plate. This was Canada's premier horse racing event, part of their own triple crown. That night we ventured down to Toronto's gay village. It took us five modes of transport to get to the village. a shuttle from the motel to the airport; then the 192 bus to the Kipling subway station, then the green line to St George station, we switched to the yellow line down to Union station, then the ancient transport of walking until we decided to take a cab as my feet were killing me in my heels. I just had to stop at a shop and purchase flip flops for comfort. Heels in the bag we made our way to the village by Church Street. The first visit was to the adult store for a browse then to a bar with drag queens on stage. The next bar I tried to enter I was immediately stopped and refused entrance as it was for males only. Well, that discrimination just made my day. My DJs had suggested I should have shown my male parts and would have got an immediate way of passage.

We settled down on a corner bar and the patio drinking an awesome cocktail which contained watermelon juice. A few pitchers later we were enjoying ourselves. Dave soon struck up a conversation with a mother and daughter at the table next to us. The mother from Germany was visiting her daughter who had been living in Toronto for the past six years. We soon learned that the mother was trying to come to terms with her daughter being a lesbian. When the daughter learned that I was not just a transgender woman, but interested in women. I could see her eyes light up with an interest in me. I had

160

just smoked a joint which I had discovered was my aphrodisiac. Sitting there at the corner cafe watching the beautiful women pass by. I felt the tingling wet sensation between my legs. I did not get an erection but felt the wetness inside of my penis. At that moment I realized how a beautiful it was to feel aroused in a female way.

We had to leave as we made our five modes of transport to make it back to the motel before the last bus from Kipling to the airport. Only to discover from the bus driver on the way back we could have caught one single bus from the airport all the way to the gay village. The next day we had a spectacular day at the Queen's Plate. We even had our photos taken on the red carpet. I was a bit disappointed as we were expecting to see Queen Elizabeth II. But instead, it was the Governor General in her place. I managed to have a few wins with at 30:1 outsider and to end the day before departing catching an exactor which helped pay for a late lunch.

A few weeks later the four of us once again recorded another unscripted show at Dave's apartment. I was feeling a bit down that Sunday as my son had canceled on our lunch get together. I knew I had to snap out of my down state so I called up my DJ's and said to them, "Let's do a show." I quickly jumped in my car and drove over to my DJ's place; Alison joined us for the show. Dave's dining room table made a perfect setting for the show. Just five minutes before we had no idea what we would discuss, after a few minutes of throwing ideas around we decided on "Tight Budgets" as all four of us were going through tough financial times like so many people. The show went off so well.

July 17, 2013, arrived marking one year as Lisa. This called for a celebration at the Cats Caboose in St Catharines. Tammy had driven down and planned to spend the night at my place. This was a night I wanted to let loose and enjoy myself. So it meant leaving my car at Cats and taking a cab back to the Falls. That afternoon Tammy and I headed out to my salon for my 6pm hair appointment with Gabriella. I arrived to see Gia, Doris, and Gabriella preparing their own hair for my party. I wanted to try something different, so Gabriella placed a purple feather extension on my right side.

Next, I had to drive over to Liz as she had volunteered to do my makeup. But as we were driving over the dark clouds were forming. There was a severe thunderstorm watch for the Niagara area. Liz had two of her male friends over. They were two great guys, Chris an actor and Nick, a hairdresser. They spent almost an hour doing my makeup and fixing my hair with extensions. When they were done, I finally saw my reflection in the mirror. All I could say was "WOW" "WOW" "WOW." What an amazing job that Liz and Nick did. I have never seen my eyes so beautiful.

By this time the storm had hit, as soon as there was a break in the weather we headed off to Cats Caboose later for my own party. Considering the severe storm seventeen of my great friends showed. We had absolutely a great time, I having so many shots that my friends kept buying for me. I was drinking Coors light but with the mixture of a martini, tequila, Goldschlager and some other shot I knew this was a recipe for a heavy hangover. On the way back home we joined Vee for a few drink at the new Latin flavor club Mojitos. Oh, what a beautiful night it was and sure as hell, I had one mean hangover the next day.

The last week in July for some reason tested my womanly strength. To stand up to men, that would prey or take advantage of women's vulnerability. The week started by a young woman entering my life through a good friend of mine. At the young age of eighteen her strong sexual desires had drawn her into the sex business. She had made the mistake that many young women who enter the sex trade make. These women would trust their lives to a pimp who was able to woo them under false promises and false security. Only to be taking advantage of, these women keeping their hard-earned money for themselves. Destiny had brought this woman to me; I had to free her from the chains of her oppressor.

After some research through my various contacts, I had in the sex business. I soon learned that this man was just garbage controlling his women by idle threats. His bark, worse than his bite. My friends gave me good advice on how she could break the chains. She must ignore all the threats and avoid any contact or replies to his constant texts and calls. Maybe it was the motherhood growing inside of me that made me take her under my wing. I had to look after my kitten as I would call her. She was drawn to me by my positive and interesting take on life.

Experiencing different cultures of the many years and meeting open-mindedly with people from all works of life. This had earned me my degree in the knowledge of life. I made her promise not to respond and stand strong; she is a woman worthy of her integrity.

With my life change and freedom gave birth to a brave new woman. A woman that had no fears not even a fear of death. I would stand up to any challenge that faces me with vigor strength. A few days later I would stand up for my Kitten once again after a male friend of mine had said some nasty words about her over a dispute on a laptop. Fury exploded inside of me as I heard the derogatory words over the phone. At that time I was with Kitty at the tattoo shop as she had her new tattoo sized up. I had to leave the building my voice rising to a higher decibel while still trying to maintain my feminine voice. No man has the right to threaten or say harsh words to a defenseless woman. I screamed back at him that I will not permit any bodily harm to a woman, even though I knew he would not follow through on the idle threats. With our friendship in ruins, he was able to reach out to me and make amend our friendship after I had uttered the words,"I have no respect for any man who threatens or does physical harm to any woman."

Next was to stand up to men in the business. A man thinking he could fool me on into machines I had purchased for my vending business. He had told me that the machines were upgraded to take the new coins in circulation when they were not. I blatantly call the man telling him he has to pay me the $100 cost for the upgrades. He passively agreed to pay me.

It took over one year when that dreaded day arrived. I would experience my first harassment as a transgender woman when I was out with my BFF Dee on a Thursday night. We headed down the newly opened Gay and Lesbian club in the Falls. Only to find it was empty, so we headed to Mints across the street. Mints was one of the few Strip Clubs that cater to both males and females offering male dancers downstairs and female dancers on the main level. Well, Dee and I were only interested in the women dancers. We sat at the bar happy to see that they had $3.75 beers on Thursday night. A good saving from their normal price of $5.50.

We struck up an interesting conversation with a beautiful dark hair dancer named Tiffany. Most of her body was cover with tattoos, with the exception of her torso. An area she had decided to keep tattoo free. Earlier that night Dee and I had -further bonded as we both realized how much more we had in common. Most of important of all we had the same taste in woman. Tiffany was just such a woman, women with tattoos was a turn on for both us women.

Dee wanted to get some cigarettes which meant leaving the club and finding a convenience store to buy the smokes. I saw down Main Street that there was a store. But as we approached closer to the store I realized we had to pass by a bar with a group of males standing outside. Instinct did tell me this could not be good. I said to myself I have the right to walk through them to get to the store. I was wearing a dress that I was I was not totally happy with as it does not compliment my body. I had found that certain tops, skirts or dresses could give the enhanced appearance of my narrow hips.

We passed by the men without an incident, but on the return, one of the men with short brown hair rushed up to me placing his face in front of mine. For a moment I thought it was someone that might have known me so I paused staring him directly into his eyes. When I realized I did not know him, I stepped aside him to pass by. He grabbed my arm saying, "Can I ask you something." There was no fear in me so I turned around to confront him. "I want to see you sometime."

I responded with a smile and turned to walk on. He followed me with his friends playing spectators to this unfolding. "I have another question for you," he said.

Immediately Dee sensing from her own harassment for being a lesbian a few times, sternly said to him, "Back off buddy." Surprisingly he did back off. I had to admit I was curious to what that second question was, even though I knew what he wanted to ask me. But I did question it in my mind was it the transgender curiosity or wishful thinking that he thought I was Dee' lesbian lover. Dee had done a great job on my makeup that night. Not deterred by the incident we walked on Later that night it dawned on me, that it was totally disrespectable on how he approached me. I am a woman in her early fifties and him possibly in his twenties. I was not one of his peers he could have fun with.

Ontario had just passed a new law making it a hate crime to discriminate or harass a transgender person. So the next day I decided to call the police as I thought it was time for someone to stand up to bullies. They had informed me that I should have called them that night so they could have responded immediately. Dee comforted me saying not to let it bug me as this might be the first in over one year, but for sure won't be the last. Even though I might be totally passable as a woman, one day I face discrimination or harassment as I am a lesbian.

It was a Wednesday night I was hanging out with Dee on my patio. We had just had a full day's work doing the vending at Niagara-On-The-Lake. It was time to relax with an ice cold beer and a treat, which I refer to as my meds. Officially diagnosed with arthritis, I could qualify for medicinal marijuana. Both of us suffering from joint pain we had the right to enjoy some weed. The subject of vaginas came up in the discussion as it could be a good topic for my next show. But the funny part was that when I had to text a friend about the idea for a show. With both our vast knowledge about vaginas, we both did not know how to spell VAGINAS. Thanks to spell check I was able to get the correct spelling.

After a long discussion about the fact that I always wanted to venture back in the local bar across the street, where Lee would frequent. It was decided I would pick up my courage and enter the lion's den. When we arrived, there were just two customers that I did recognize, but neither one recognized me. Eventually, after a few drinks, I spoke to the barmaid who I had known not too well. She did acknowledge she did recognize me and was totally cool about it. Soon after two women entered the bar, the older a black woman and the younger woman of mixed race she was cold from the chill outside. So Dee offered the younger woman her denim jacket a gesture well appreciated by her. Soon after we struck up conversations with them. They moved down the bar to be closer to us. Ella mentioned she was thirty-three years old, so I responded that I was just one year old. Her interest in me spiked when I started telling her about my transgender transition. Both women were not aware that I was a transgender woman, boosting myself esteem to higher levels. Ella was quick to mention that she was bisexual and that she was so turned on by me. At that point, Dee and Barb went out for a cigarette. We were both left alone in the bar with the exception of a group of four who were across the bar at the table. and the barmaid. She turned around to me and said: "what the hell let's do it." We embraced each other our parted lips joining in unbridled passion. Tongues exploring each other warm mouths. She paused for a moment telling me, "I can be either masculine or feminine. I want to throw you down and make love to you." What a wonderful moment that reassured me that there are women out there that will be attracted to a transgender woman. I had to embrace the fact that I am rare human species that is, who would have lived as both genders. We left off with the intent we will hook up soon to experience our lust for each other.

10 August 2013, Saturday

D-Day had finally arrived. After much soul searching and asking advice from friends. I finally reached the decision to tell my aging parents about my transition. Most of my friends had advised against this, with the exception of three very close friends: Harry, Dee, and Di. All three had suggested I follow my heart and tell my parents. I made a quick call to my sister Alyson as I had just spoke to her on the phone a week before. Emotionally I had told her it was eating at my insides I had to tell the folks. If she could discuss the matter with my other two sisters. The thought of "it will kill them if you tell them" was the constant family theme. But my response was always, "If they heard it from another source and not me. That would kill them. "In the back of my mind I had worried, what if I had told them and one of them dies of a heart attack. My whole family will hold it against me. But my gut feeling was telling me that this would not be the case.

At about 12pm South African time I received the green light from Alyson. They had discussed it and came to the conclusion that I must do what I feel is best. It was suggested that I call them about 1pm when they would arrive back home from a family barbecue at Alyson's house. 1pm approached nervously I went to the bathroom. I needed to do number two; the thought of me shitting myself was real. All of a sudden my electronic doorbell rang. I rushed over to the door to see who it was. But there was nobody there. Was this a spiritual sign telling me it was time to face the music?

I put on my Skype headphones and made the anticipated call. It rang a few times then my Dad answered the phone. "Is Mom there as well?" I would normally have both of them on the line with their two phone system. My niece Cindy was there to support them if needed. She had casually made it look like she was just over for a visit. With both of them on the phone, I made sure that they were both sitting down. I proceeded to tell them they must promise not to worry about what I have to tell them. Only after I got the verbal agreement from them, I proceeded to tell them about my GID (gender identity dysphoria). The word disorder now replaced with dysphoria in the medical term. The idea was just to tell them this part that day. I was supposed to hold back the part that I had actually started the transition.

To my pleasant surprise, they took it so well. Even my father commenting that it was good that I had told them. I asked if they were okay with me to proceed, which they both agreed. Telling them that I had started the true life test, my transition had begun with hormones and therapy. Most important of all that I was so happy and free to finally be myself. I ended the conversation telling them that even if they don't understand my actions. They must at least be happy for me as I am finally free and truly happy. If they had any questions, they must be free to ask any. My Dad said he would make note of any questions they might have for my next conversation. I closed the phone feeling the final weight finally lifted off my shoulders. Knowing well that my folks might experience an aftershock from this revelation.

As expected there were aftershocks the week that followed. I received an angry email from my brother as I had not consulted him before telling the folks. He also commented, "*I for one will not be looking at your You Tube videos because I don't think that it respects where we are at all, and the grandstanding is out of place.*" That spurred a quick retaliation email from me stating, On the point of "grandstanding is out of place." You will never be able to understand the freedom and happiness that I can finally be myself. So it is not grandstanding as you stay but the feeling of finally not having to live with the burden I carried for all these years. I do apologize for trying to reach out to you as a brother."

Other emails from my sisters followed with their soothing words to calm the situation down. *"We are family, and we should all try not to make things worse for mom and dad by using harsh words when we communicate with each other. The discussions around these e-mails tear my immediate family apart, and life is too short for that."*

One week later I called them for my follow up call. But this call would be different, now I was free to be Lisa. But when I heard the tone from my mother and father I could sense that they were still in shock of the news. Even though the first call had gone well, it was seeping into their minds they had lost their son. My father's words to me were very consoling to me. "I just want to let you know that we still love you, this does not change our love for you. "I could not help but feel the sense of joy, unconditional love ruled the day.

That night I had four of my girlfriends over for a ladies night. This would be my first slumber party. Just a few days earlier I had come to the realization that I was going through my puberty as a girl. Was that the reason why I was connecting to women from all age groups from eighteen to fifty? I was experiencing a crash course on becoming a woman. Kitty was my link to the late teen years I am missed, never being that little girl growing up to be a woman. It did not bother me that I had lost all that opportunity to experience the life of a girl. What is important in now, the present. I am living the life I meant to be, happy and free as a woman. The words of **Simone de Beauvoir** would become my new motto:

172

"One is not born, but rather becomes, a woman."

Sunday morning I saw the email from my brother. I was afraid to read it, I did not want any negativity to pull me down after a wonderful night with my closest female friends. I had posted the comment with the group photo. *"Thank you to all my beautiful angels for the awesome night."* That afternoon I picked up the courage to read the email. To my pleasant surprise, it was a consolatory reply with an apology. I replied back with a consolatory email explaining that with the hormones came the change of emotions.

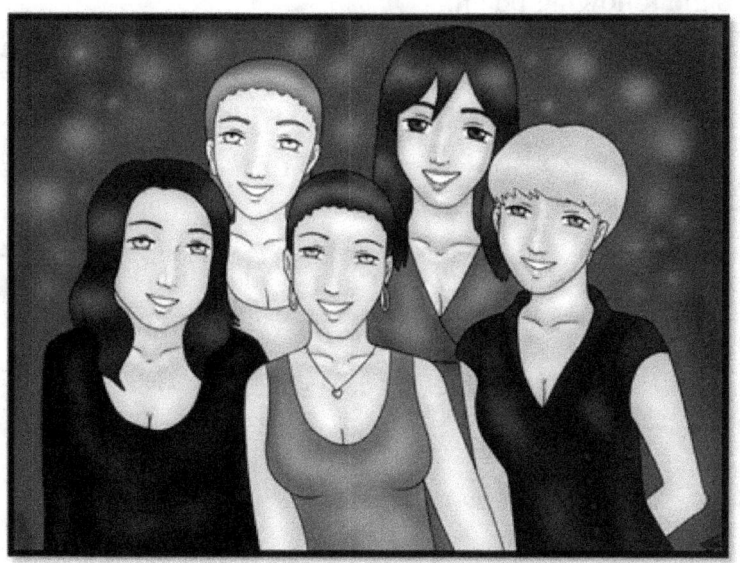

Figure 13 Slumber Party 2013 Dee, Sylvia, Tammy, Lisa & Victoria

173

Chapter Nine

Vagina Envy

During one of our regular discussions on my patio, where we would have a few beers at the occasional joint. Dee made a very interesting comment. "Once you have had the operation, you will no longer be diagnosed as GID (gender identity dysphoria). At that point, you will be just a woman." I so longed for that day when I can finally have my vagina. She would always say to me that she too longs for the day when I don't have to tell anyone that I am transgender. But instead just a regular woman. My desire for my vagina-inspired me to write the following poem:

When I Get My Vagina
by Lisa Alexandra

Happiness rules the day
Trees hosts chirping birds
The white dove above flying free
Butterflies emerge from their cocoons
Mind and body are finally in sync
The bud becomes the rose

No more ball ache

174

No more concealing
Silk caresses the skin
A smooth frontier between the legs
Nylons embrace my limbs
A new awakening of female joy
Sensual comforting and stimulating

I walk along the water's edge
the gentle salty waves caress my feet
The ivory skirt swaying in the wind
My body touched by the breeze
Hair flowing freely in the breeze
I dance and twirl in total bliss
No weight between my thighs

I stare out at sea
I am finally the woman
I meant to be.

In October Dee and I became roommates. For a while, I was contemplating finding a roommate for my spare bedroom to help with my financial situation. This was a good solution for both of as we get on so well. Besides our strong friendship, we both complement each other. We both have our kids grown up and have moved out of the home. I noticed that women take it harder when their kids finally leave the nest. For me, it was my moment to start my transition, but for mothers, it is a trying time to cut the strings. Dee is such a help in advising me on how to dress, what clothes to buy. Having two beautiful daughters of her own, she was skilled in choosing the right clothes to compliment one's body. I have submitted to her choice in clothing. We have opted to go for the classier feminine look. It is amazing how the right clothing mix of colors and designs can help transform you into a beautiful woman. Now that winter was upon us, I had worn more jeans or long pants.

Winter does bring a bit more pain as I have to secure myself in the crotch wearing two panties. The testicle pain only validates my desire to have them removed. I did seriously consider the intermediate surgery of removing my testicles, an operation referred to as orchiectomy or orchi for short. It is not a complicated surgery that only leaves a small insertion scar where they enter to remove the testicles. The operation can even be done in an outpatient facility. A local anesthetic is used. The penis is taped to the abdomen. A small incision is made in the middle of the scrotum. The testicles are removed, and the spermatic cord is cut.

I research the pros and cons of having an orchi. The pros were that I could stop taking Spiroton the male blocker; I would have a smoother crotch and no more testicle pain. The cons were that if I wait too long for the GRS, the scrotum skin will shrink. The scrotum skin is a very important part that is used in creating the vagina lips. I decided to contact Dr. Brassard's office in Montreal to get their opinion on the matter. I was pleasantly surprised to receive a rapid reply the next day. It was recommended for me to wait for my GRS. As they prefer to remove the testicles during the operation. For me having an orchi would have felt like a half measure. From a psychological, I would prefer to wait and go for the surgery. Knowing well that the outcome, I would finally a full woman.

The thought of me finally having my vagina did bring on some naughty thoughts. Even though I am only attracted to females. I do feel the desire to take my vagina for a test ride. I fantasize about being the slut for a day, week or so. In one of our Sex Talk shows Bella explained it in a meaningful way, "you want your vagina penetrated by men as a validation that you are finally a physically and emotionally a woman."

Three months had passed that I have not seen my son. We stayed in communication through texting and the occasional call. My worry is that when he finally sees me, I will be totally a different person. Lee is fading rapidly, and I feel my personality is so much in tune of that of a woman's. No longer will he see the father in me. There are times I cry alone missing the closeness that my son and I had. But knowing well I am on the path of no return.
My friend Harry from Australia even made a comment to me that it was like starting up a new friendship relationship with me as Lisa.

Lee was dead and gone, never to return. My physical appearance has changed so vastly, breasts forever slowly growing, hair growing past my shoulders. My personality is that of the woman, Lisa.

The work day was done 21 November 2013; I was on the elevator to my condo when the phone rang. I scrambled to find my phone in my bag. Grasping the phone, I saw the "private number" caller ID answering as quickly as I could.

"Hi I am calling for Lisa." Was the female voice on the other end.

"This is Lisa." I replied.

"I am Candice from the Gender Identity Clinic in Toronto."

Joy and excitement overwhelmed me, as we approached my floor. She went on to explain she was doing follow up calls to all the transgender people whose first assessment was approaching. She wanted to know how everything was going with my transgender journey.

I was quick to explain I had reached the mental and physical state of no return. No one and as harsh as it may sound, not even my son would make me revert back to my old male life. I was totally committed waiting anxiously for that day I could have my surgery to complete my journey. I went on to explain the testicle pain I experience, even more so with the winter months approaching. I was wearing jeans more often. It meant I had to secure my penis and testicles even more to create the smooth crotch. This was achieved by wear two panties. I would try wearing longer tops to cover my crotch area. I explained I had researched the option of having my testicles removed. I had concluded with the help of the advice from the GRS clinic in Montreal. That I will wait for my final operation. She said that this could possibly help in moving me up the waiting list. By the end of the conversation, I was informed that I will only require one assessment as opposed to the recommended two. I was ready to start my discussions on my surgery. There would be another meeting after the assessment sometime before the surgery. She requested that I send two professional references that showed I was operating my vending company as Lisa.

Immediately after I closed the phone, extremely happy I worked on the two references. I obtained one from my bank and the other from the vending supplier from St Catharines that I deal with. That very same day I emailed the two references along with the poem I had written "When I Get my Vagina."

Chapter Ten

The fairy Appears

December 5, 2013, was a day that would be marked down in history. On this day the world received news of Nelson Mandela's death. This was a passing that was anticipated yet mourned by so many people around the world. His death inspired me to write this Facebook post:

I cannot forget the country that gave me birth: South Africa. I salute a man of courage, conviction, passion, wisdom and reconciliatory. A truly great man Nelson Mandela RIP Madiba. I am proud to know that I share a bond with this remarkable man. Both born males in South Africa, both imprisoned for many years. His the chains of oppression, mine chains of the male body.

Another woman had entered my life prior to this day. Christine a twenty-seven year old blonde, mother of four. Petite in size, yet enormous in character. We met at a mutual friend's party, a masquerade post-Halloween, Master Blaze and Mistress Avaya. Mistress Avaya made all the masks herself an awesome creative job, to say the least. A roof was built over the outdoor bar they called Swaggerville. Sheets of canvas hung to prevent the cold fall breeze from entering. In the middle of the bar, stood a tall gas heater, radiating warmth into the bar.

I had secured my spot at the end of the bar, vodka and punch in my hand. I looked up to see this petite cute blond appear in front of me. Like a fairy with just her wings missing. Shortly into our conversations which took an immediate interest in the transgender subject. We both knew we were meant to meet that day. She commented she almost did not come to the party in fear that she would not know too many people. But realized she was meant to come that day, destiny had led our path to cross. Her hippy approach to life had intrigued me. With the vodka flowing and six joints later, we indulged in an in depth interesting conversation. She was part native Indian, a trait that would always draw me to that person.

A week or two had past when we finally reconnected through Facebook. It was a Thursday night that we would meet up at her house in the Falls. We smoked a joint in her bathroom, before heading out to her friend's cocktail Christmas party at her spa. Dressed for the occasion Dee, Christine and I entered the spa. Sandy had done her own unique design of the studio using mostly black and white. Sandy was a beautiful, dark-haired, slim woman that possessed both style and class. She was dressed in a black outfit her friendly manner led me to purchased one of her two for one vouchers. I settled for a relaxing massage and pedicure voucher.

The next days that followed by Christine present in my life by meeting over at each other respective house for a visit. After a few attempts I finally able to make the appointment for the relaxing massage followed by a pedicure. The massage to its description very relaxing and calming, light music playing in the candle lit room. Arriving home, I was greeted by a delicious roast beef dinner by Dee. After pacing back on forth, it was agreed that along with Sandy, Christine, and some other friends. That we will venture to Mints, the male and female strip club.

That we all meet t Mints, the upstairs part of course, where all the female dancers were.

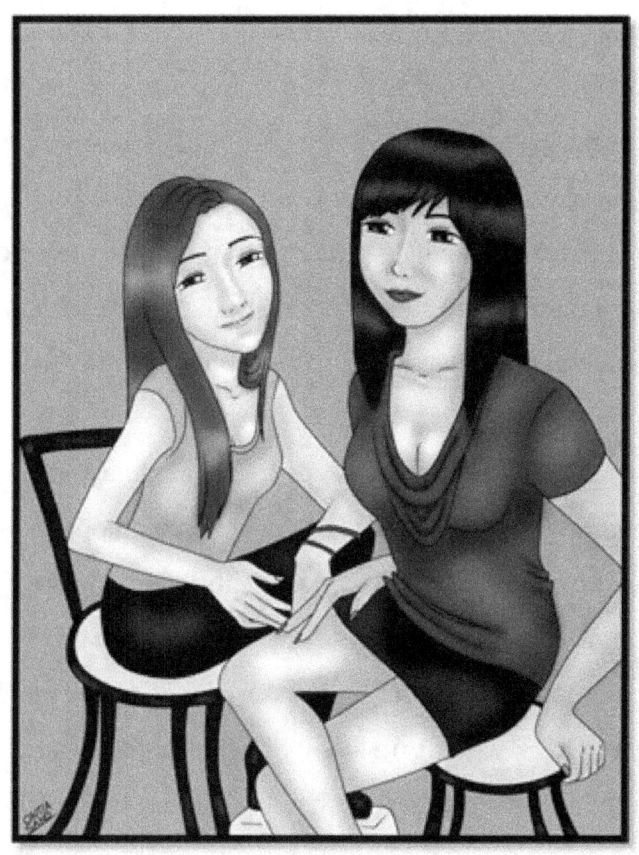

Figure 14 Christine & Lisa

Here is an Email I received from Harry after I had sent him some pictures from the past. Titled: "Blast from the Past". His response was a question that does plague my mind.

"*Thanks for the memories. So you reminiscing? Makes me sad and wonder. What do you do with all the memories and pics of Lee. Surely he will always be remembered. Do you remember Lee as a third person or is it psychologically complex and you remember him as yourself*".

My response, "I do tend to speak about Lee as a third person. Dee kept calling me on the fact that I refer to Lee as a third person. So I refer to it as **my past life**. I do feel a bit out of place when I am with a bunch of women, and they were talking about their past. I never go to experience growing up as a girl. The past is part of me I do cherish those moments in the past. Amsterdam and Germany will always remain good memories with awesome friends. Lisa"

14 January 2014, Tuesday 10:24 pm: The next day was the day I had been waiting for so long. Finally my first and hopefully my deciding assessment with the Gender Identity Clinic were upon me. I was expecting, or I should say was hoping to get the transgender female psychologist. But instead, I was assigned to the male doctor. Remembering back when I first visited a psychologist back in Durban in my twenties. I recalled her saying that I would have had to have one session with a male and female doctor on separate occasions. So I looked at it positively. I have skipped the first assessment with the possibility of this been seen as my second. Earlier on during the day I had prepared all the papers needed. Then went into preparing for my so called pitch speech:

   1. **One Year Real-life Test:** I applaud the transgender protocol for making this a requirement. For me, it only reconfirmed my commitment and desire to forge forward to become the woman I meant to be.

2. **Conviction No turning back:** I am finally becoming the true person I meant to be LISA., would not even turn back for my son. Brett who is warming up to accepting me as a transgender person.

3. **I will not miss my Penis**: a recent time with a female friend. I had sex with her both as a male role with the help of Viagra. Then having sex as a woman to woman. I confirmed I will not miss my penis. As I have started experiencing the female orgasm without an erection.

4. **Testicle Pain:** Having to tuck and conceal my genitals, I have to deal with testicle pain constantly. After research on a possible orchi. I looked at the pros and cons. The reply from the surgeon in Montreal helped decide for me to wait. They recommended I wait and remove my testicles at the time of the operation. Waiting another year will be torture.

5. **Support Circle:** I have not needed to continue therapy or go to support groups. I was fortunate to have the best support from my female and male friends. Especially the female friends that helped and advised me on my femininity.

15 January 2014, Wednesday
Assessment Day: Fucken Eh!

Finally, the day had arrived. Dee my wing woman by my side we headed off to Toronto. The plan was to go to Long Tall Sally, the

185

store that caters to tall women. I had set aside $200 to treat myself on some much needed tall woman's clothing. Atrium on the Bay was our destination downtown Toronto. The shopping mall also home to Red Lobster, the place we had chosen for lunch. Conveniently they had undercover parking. After squeezing into a tight parking space. We headed up the elevator to Long Tall Sally.

It so happened the 6" 3" manager's name was also Lisa. Dee helped me pick out some long sleeve tops on a special. I so needed some for the winter. Noticing that the taller store cloth sizes were different, I was able to fit into large as opposed to my regular size of XL. A red and pink top was my first items to buy. Dee made me try on a black skirt I just had to by. A tall black woman poked her head around the dressing room to see what it looked like. This was fun tall women around me, admiring each other's choices. Before leaving, I had to ignore the high prize and buy my long awaited long pink bathroom robe.

Bags in hand we headed out of the store. Only to find a store on adjacent with deals I had to buy. I was in their small dressing room cubical. Dee handing me over summer tops I just had to try on. "Hey, Dee we have to go eat" I insisted, slowly the pressure of me missing my appointment was on my mind. This was one appointment I could not risk missing. Quickly choosing the best two tops I paid and headed straight to Red lobster.

I asked the waiter how quick the food will be, as I had an important meeting to go to. Google maps had shown the CAMH building was only a 4-minute drive away. The meals came quickly. I had ordered the sole which I was not too thrilled about. Dee was happy with her pasta choice. The bill finally came; we had just 30 minutes to make it to by meeting.

We quickly paid for the parking at the machines, a costly parking of $11, but this was a special day. I had to bear whatever costs occurred that important day. Switching on my GPS, I selected the new address. Knowing well that I had to drive out of the building for the GPS to pick up the satellite. I approached the exit, no satellite signal yet. So I was faced with the choice turn left or right. I gambled on the right which turned out to be the wrong choice. The GPS finally getting the signal and pointing out I was going the wrong way. The tall building in downtown Toronto would cause the satellite to lose communication at times. Not to mention all the one-way streets causing havoc for me. Finally, I was on target finding the underground parking instructions had shown on my letter I had received. They happened to be working on some maintenance right by the parking entrance. Causing me more delay. I looked down at my watch. Just 8 minutes to my 3pm appointment. I was told to be there 10 minutes earlier to fill out some forms. I once again squeezed into a tight parking. So tight that Dee had to get out of the van before I squeezed in. Now we had to find the elevator that would take me to the 6th floor.

Finally, we found the elevator only to find out that the 6th-floor button does not work. My brain was racing. Maybe you have to go to the 7th floor and walk down as this was a secure floor? So we tried that, only to find none of the door numbers matched the door I had to find. At this point I was starting to panic, this meeting was so important to me. Five minutes to 2:50pm, I frantically ran around the corners until we found a woman who informed us that we were in the wrong building. The parking space bellow was for two building towers. We had chosen the wrong one.

At this point, I was almost in tears. Dee was trying to calm me down. Telling me not to worry, I will be on time. "You don't understand Dee, this is so important to me, I cannot miss it. Frantically I reached for my cell phone, trying to call the office that I was on the way. Finally, we were directed to the right building and up to the 6th floor. Finally arriving at the door I meant to be at, time 2:51pm. Taking a deep breath, I sat down to fill in the forms. After handing in the forms, I was given a chart and directed to my Psychologists door. The door had the sign "meeting in progress". But this was my meeting so I knocked at the door. The Doctor appeared with a student by his side. She was a young student from Asian descent about twenty years old. The Doctor asked if I was okay with the student attending the meeting. I immediately agreed that I was okay with her being present. I felt more comfortable with a female present. I was told to wait outside the door as we discussed my case in private. I took this time to gather my thoughts.

"I am ready," I told myself. Finally, the door opened, and I was invited to the small office. My seat was directly in front of the Doctor, they student facing me on the right. I opened the conversation by telling him I had a small speech planned. He graciously obliged and let me confidently state my five points. I also took this opportunity to hand him over the three personal testimonial letters that three of my closest friends had written. One was an email from Tammy; the computer typed letter from Dee and the handwritten letter from Christine. Christine and I had just become friends for only three months. In that short time, she had earned her place in my inner circle of awesome friends. The Doctor appreciated the three letters I gave to him.

At the end of the five points, he commented on my statements telling me that it showed I had put a lot of thought into my assessment. To me, he was my judge and jury, my gateway to the operation. Confidently I answered his questions starting off with my early childhood. All was going smoothly until he asked me about my puberty years. I was slightly caught off guard. My thoughts were more focused on my transgender journey over the last two tears. I am ready I kept on thinking.

I don't know how my answer went over with him. As I had replied to him that, my adolescent time was a long time ago. I don't remember my thoughts at that time. Though I do remember being happy that I could finally ejaculate at about the age of thirteen or so. I did not tell him this, focusing on the point that besides South Africa's bad apartheid past, the country was very conservative back then. Back then I could not mention or openly act of my gender diaspora.

He was happy to see that I had all my Canadian Government IDs changed into my new name. At first, he had said the fact that I was self-employed was a bit difficult to show that I was living as Lisa for my business. I presented some of my reference letters and business contracts that showed my name as Lisa.

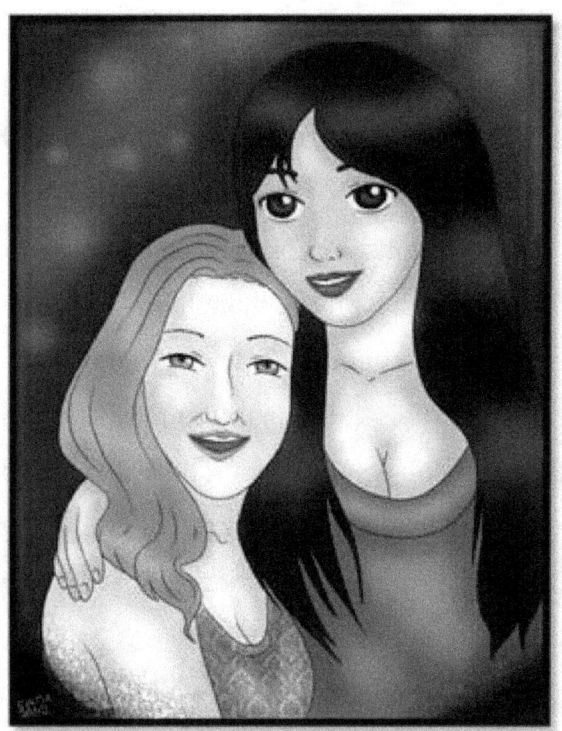

Figure 15 Tammy & Lisa

As expected he touched on the subject of suicide. He asked me if I had ever had suicidal thoughts. Vee, the transgender woman that had gone through the operation, had cautioned me about this question. I focused on telling him that I am such a positive person. When I am down, I know the only way from there is up. I held back mentioning the dark memory of that near-fatal day at Sun City when I came close to taking my life. That moment was not part of me now. Never again did I ever fall to that low since that day, which gave me my strength to carry on.

I had earlier emailed my social worker that I needed the letter from the Doctor for my Dutch passport name and gender. This request was passed on to him, so I reminded him about it.

Gender change surgery-man transforms into a female

Then came the most important question of all!

"What does the operation mean for you? Why do you feel you need it."

Think back at what Vee had replied to me, when I asked her a few months after her operation, "How do you feel now, do you miss your penis?" Her response forever branded in my brain.

"It just feels right." Was her response back then.

So my reply was, "I will finally feel complete, my mind and body will be in sync. This is what would make me a complete woman"

Feeling confident I had stated my case.

At the end, he wrote a handwritten letter for the Dutch courts for my passport change. I had to correct him as he first wrote my old name "Lee." I pointed out to him that I was now Lisa. He informed me that it will take about six weeks before I get his report through my Doctor.

This special day had brought about many positive developments prior to the day. My Dutch lawyer had asked if I wanted to proceed with the case. I had finally got the last two documents needed for the 10 March court hearing in the Haag, for my make and gender request.

Now I even had the handwritten letter from the psychologist. Stating that I met the medical criteria for gender dysphoria. A diagnose is very important in the steps of being approved for the GRS surgery. But the sad thing was that I had no more funds to continue paying the lawyers. Even though we were so close to finalizing the documents required. So I took the chance of asking her if there was any chance of legal aid. She sent me a link to a pro-bono lawyer. To my surprise, I had a response to my request I had sent online.

Within a few weeks, I was approved for the pro-bono lawyer. My old lawyer had said I might not qualify as I don't live in the Netherlands. But as fate would have it my pro-bono female Lawyer came to my rescue. It so turned out that she is passionate about helping the LGTB community, donating some of her free time. Giving anti-bulling speeches at school. She acknowledged to me that she was in fact married to a woman. This connection made me happy. Here was a woman that has never met me and knows very little about me. Came to my rescue to fight for my right to be recognized as a woman.

Counting the days that following my assessment, six weeks had passed. So I emailed CAMH asking how my report was proceeding. Reminding them of my testicle pain, that would hopefully speed up the process. The next day I received the reply:

I just forwarded your email to Dr. B**** so he is aware of your request to include your pain in his report. Dr. Baici has prepared your report, but we are just waiting to case conference it. We anticipate being able to do so on March 11th or 18th. I will call you after the case conference to inform you what the next steps are. I apologize for the delay.

and my reply

Thanks for the update. I so look forward to your call after the case conference. I am hoping and praying it will be the words "You are approved for the Operation!"

Thanks
Lisa

So I waited passionately for two important outcomes. Finally, the 18th March arrived. Sitting at my computer on a Skype call I heard my phone ring. Looking down that the caller ID showing "Unknown number". I knew this has to be CAMH and so I excused myself urgently from my Skype call.

It was Chrissie the words, "There must have been a misunderstanding about the one assessment. You do need one more assessment, but you are on the list for surgery approval." This was not the words I was expecting, but as the positive person, I am I took it as a positive. In the back of my mind, I knew I had to have two physiologists sign off for my operation. I was told that my next CAMH meeting should be within six weeks. At this point in my journey, I was used to *waiting.......*

17 April 2014, Thursday
My HERO delivers

I woke up to my regular routine, freshening up, brushing my teeth, etc.. Every day with the same thought "ok what excuse can I use to get out of doing my exercises? I have a busy day today. I have a hangover. I'm in a rush I don't have time to do my exercises." But without failing, I will force myself.

I would start with jumping jacks to warm up. Then lying on the carpet on the left side of my bed, I would do two sets of twenty stomach crunches. Followed by lying on my back and lifting my legs

194

in the air. Parting them as wide as possible. I learned this from a girlfriend you will soon be introduced to. As a yoga instructor, I had asked her how can I train my legs to part like a woman's? As you know, women can spread their legs a lot wider than most men. If the curious need arises to have sex with a man or a woman for that matter. I would like to be able to spread the legs like a natural born female. Using my twelve-pound weights, I would end off with three sets of squats. An exercise well needed as I had to re-strengthen my legs so that I could squat down to pick up things like a woman. Next was to make my milk coffee, I got accustomed to the café latte while living in the Caribbean. I sat down at my desk placing the coffee next to me. I switched on the computer monitor wiggling the mouse to wake up the computer. Every morning I would check my email using Microsoft Outlook. My eye immediately caught the attention of the email from my pro-bono Lawyer. It read:

Dear Lisa,

Welcome to the world of women!

Hereby the verdict of the Dutch court. It is agreed that both your name and gender will be changed on your birth certificate, and as such in your passport.

But: there is a three month period for the state (and for us) to register an appeal.

After that date, the verdict will be registered. In July you can go and get your new passport.

Congratulations, and thanks for the trust in me.
Sophia.

Overwhelmed with joy, I jumped up running to Dee in the kitchen. Tears of joy flooding to my eyes I informed Dee of the wonderful news. This was one of my biggest mountains I had to climb. There was a time when I almost gave up on trying to change my name and gender on my Dutch passport. My determination and refusing to give up and most important of all my hero finally paid off. A few days later still excited by the news I sent Sophia an email.

Dear Sophia

My transgender journey as beautiful as it is. Has had its tough moment. The fight to change my name and gender has been one of my biggest mountains I had to climb. With my gender change came a major financial change. Making me start all over again, to fight my way back to the top. Today was a beautiful moment when I received your email.

Sophia, you are my HERO. *A Hero I have never met or even know what you look like. You who did not know too much about me, so graciously took on my case. To fight not only for what is right but what has granted me my freedom rights. The right to be **finally recognized as a woman**. Truly a beautiful day all due to your conviction and belief in helping the LGTB community.*

I am truly indebted to you. I hope that someday I can repay you the joy you have given to me.

One happy woman
Lisa

Chapter Eleven

Reality Sinks In

Through Christine, another woman entered into my life. Samantha was a beautiful tall, slim woman with a toned body, dark hair. We had met at her open house of her spa she had owned. The spa was done in a classy She had immediately caught my attention by her classy demeanor. We spoke briefly that night, even though money was tight I found myself under her spell. Purchasing one of her 2 for 1 certificate for a massage and manicure.

We entered the candlelit massage room, soft music playing in the background. I asked politely "Excuse me for asking this but do I strip down completely?" She was aware that I was a transgender woman and was totally comfortable giving me a massage. Samantha replied that it was up to me and that I could go totally naked as I will be covered by the towels.

As the massage began with me face down a naughty memory came back to me. In the Caribbean, I had learned that if the masseuse starts you off on your stomach, it could mean that a "happy ending" was possible. I felt so comfortable in her presence. I told her about this supposed Caribbean rule. She laughed informing me it was definitely not one of those massages. The ice was cracked as I found myself being very open and honest with her. In return, she opened up a bit of her interesting life. This day was the birth of a great new friendship. Two intelligent, independent business women slightly with mischievous minds. Samantha had become the close girlfriend that girls would have growing up experiencing puberty together. I now had a smart, beautiful sexy woman advising me dress tips to makeup. We would hang out on my girl like school girls, chatting about boys, business, and other crazy subjects.

We were destined to do something together. Thus becoming business partners in our new venture with Back alley Apps. This company would focus purely on developing apps for the adult market. Thus giving us both the opportunity to put our naughty sides to use.

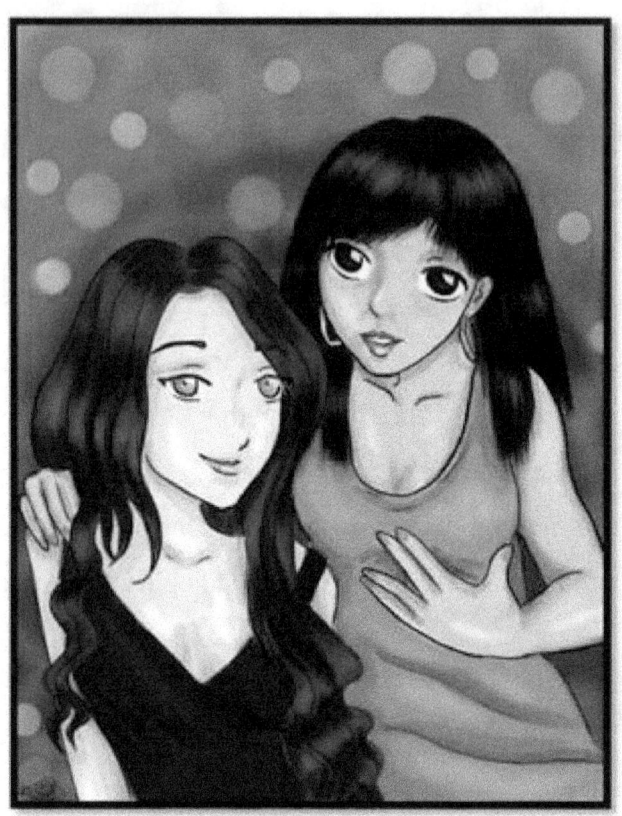

Figure 16 Samantha & Lisa

On the 30th of April, I finally received my appointment for my surgery approval assessment. Scheduled for the 14th of May at 2pm. I was to be on two assessments, one from the same psychologist that saw me the first time and the social worker Christina. The days leading up to this important day were extremely busy for me as I had more machine installations to do for my vending business.

Along with the busy work schedule, the realization that I was finally coming closer to my dream of becoming a full woman was sinking in. In preparation for the assessments, I had to understand and be ready to discuss three very important points.

1. Understanding the whole MTF surgery procedure referred to as vaginoplasty.
2. Understanding the risks of the operation
3. Plans to make my way up to Montreal and plans for the aftercare of the operation.

These important points will determine my readiness for the operation. I received the link to the document that covered the three important steps. Here is part of the CAMH Trans Care Transgender Transition guide:

Vaginoplasty

The term vaginoplasty includes several procedures designed to transform the "male" genitals into "female" genitals. Usually, most of the surgery is done as one step (removing the testicles; partially removing the penis; and creating a vagina, clitoris, and labia), but some surgeons prefer to work on the labia and clitoral hood as a second stage of surgery.

In vaginoplasty, the surgeon's goals are:
• To preserve the ability to have orgasms.

201

• To create a clitoris, labia, and opening to the vagina (introitus) that look realistic and maintain good touch sensation (i.e., you can feel it when they are touched).

• To create a vagina that will hold its shape, is sensitive to touch, is wide and long enough for sexual penetration (by fingers, a dildo, or a penis), and has a moist, elastic, and hairless lining.

• To change the structures of the urinary tract so you urinate downwards and in a steady stream.

The most common technique for creating a vagina is the penile inversion. In this technique, the penis is skinned and the skin is turned inside out to line the walls of the new vagina. In some cases, extra skin is required to make the vagina longer or wider; this is usually taken from the lower abdomen or the scrotal sac. A segment of your large intestine may be used to create the vagina if the penile inversion fails or is not possible (e.g., because your penis was damaged or removed when you were younger). As part of the penile inversion, a small section of the head of the penis – the part that is most sensitive – is used to create a new clitoris. Erectile tissue, which gives the penis the ability to get hard, will be removed so the entrance to the vagina and the clitoris don't get overly swollen when you get sexually aroused. The tube that carries urine from the bladder to the outside of the body (urethra) is longer in "males" than in "females," and in a slightly different position. The urethra is shortened and repositioned as part of vaginoplasty. The prostate *(which sits at the neck of the bladder, around the urethra) is not removed. The innermost labia (labia minora) are typically made from leftover skin from the penis. The outer labia (labia majora) are usually made from testicle skin. Revisions are sometimes needed after vaginoplasty to refine the appearance of the labia, as well as the clitoris or its hood.*

Risks and possible complications of MTF genital surgery

Possible complications specific to vaginoplasty include:
• fistula: opening between the rectum and new vagina
• decreased sexual sensation, and possible decreased ability to have orgasm
• partial or total death of the tissue used to create the new vagina, labia, or clitoris
• narrowing or closure of the new vagina or urethra
• prolapse: vagina falling out of the body
• hair growth in the vagina (from hair-bearing tissue used as vaginal lining)
• unsatisfactory size or shape of the new vagina, clitoris, or labia

Extracted from Trans Care Project, February 2006 Vancouver Coastal Health, Transcend Transgender Support & Education Society and Canadian Rainbow Health Coalition

Sitting down on the toilet a few days later I found myself staring down at my penis. "You will soon be gone; we had some good times together." I said in my mind. The thought of the extreme evasive surgery was sinking in. It was hard to say if I was nervous or feared what was coming. I thought of Jesus before his crucifixion. Jesus knew it was coming, feared it but knew it had to happen. There was no doubt what I wanted or any second thought of me backing out. There was no stopping destiny, I would have my vagina.

Mother's day arrived just a few days before my appointment. I called up my mom in South Africa to wish her happy Mother's Day. To my pleasant surprise she addressed me as Lisa for the very first time. One simple gesture, one giant heartwarming moment. This immediately put me at ease to discuss with my mom the upcoming appointment and about the actual surgery. Mother's Day 2014 will always be remembered as a beautiful day.

That evening Vee and her roommate stopped by for a visit. She arrived with a beautiful red bouquet of flowers for Mother's day. This was a perfect time for me to question Vee about her operation, now that two years had passed. I was so happy to hear that her vagina is fully functional. She has feelings internally and stimulation feeling on her clitoris. It took her six months to experience her first post op orgasm. The other point I discussed was my plans to return home after my operation. Driving back was ruled out as I can expect to feel tired and could not stay in the car too long. My next options were to either fly or catch the train back home.

14 May 2014, Wednesday

Surgery Approval Assessment

My morning was hectic, trying to take care of important administration for my business. My two besties Christine and Dee came to my rescue. They would take care of the vending that day. While transferring the products from my van to Christine's van. I told her that I was feeling a bit stressed about the appointment. My mind was so busy with taking care of business that I did not give myself time to quietly reflect and prepare for the upcoming appointment.

This day was extremely important to me. This is the appointment that would lead to my surgery approval. Was I ready for this? Christine calmly said to me "Lisa don't worry we will take care of the business. Just focus on your appointment, you got this one babe." Her words gave me peace of mind for a moment.

Samantha had accompanied me on the trip to Toronto. On the way to pick her up the ever so long train in Niagara Falls had broken down. Causing a major delay, as it was obstructing my route to pick up Samantha. I could not risk waiting for the train On Drummond Rd to move. So I drove up to the QEW in a roundabout way to pick up other bestie.

On the hour and a half drive up I explained to Samantha, how stressed out I was. Her soothing tone and interesting conversations along the way calmed me down. Arriving in Toronto I was ready for my meeting, as we were driving through Chinatown. I turned to

Samantha and said "maybe I should turn off my phone so that I don't get any text or call that would interrupt my calm demeanor"

"Just don't answer the phone," was her reply. Looking back I wished I had turned off the phone.

We had arrived a bit early so we decided to go to Tim Horton's for a light lunch. I settled for a bowl of soup and a roll. Finding a spot at the window we sat on the high chairs. The buzz of Toronto traffic outside the window. I heard my phone beep as a message came in. Out of habit I picked up the phone to see who had sent the message, it was from Dee.

As I read her message the feeling of anxiety came flooding back. It was just fifteen minutes before my appointment. She had texted me about payments for Christine. Angrily I responded to her which returned response that sent my anxiety levels even higher. At that point Samantha saw how stressed I was and took the phone away from me. So that she could wisely and calmly respond to the texts.

"Pull yourself together girl" I said to myself. "Don't let this unfortunate distraction ruin your positivity." Leaving Timmies I gave Samantha a hug as I headed up to the sixth floor for my first appointment. Samantha headed off to Chinatown to do some shopping.

Arriving on the sixth floor I bumped into my psychologist. We engaged in friendly conversation that happily had a calming effect on me. I had to wait a few minutes outside his office, so that he could review my files beforehand. Deep in thought as I sat opposite in the narrow corridor. Finally his door opened. It was time for me to shine.

Like the first assessment I had prepared a speech. Unlike my five point speech. This one was short and to the point.

"You hold the key to my future. Open the cage door and let me be the woman I'm meant to be. I am mentally and physically ready for the operation. If there is any doubt about my readiness or points of concern. Please address it today"

He proceeded in questioning me about the operation, risks and aftercare. All of which I was totally ready for. At the end he said that he will state in his report that I was ready. But there has to be a case discussion before the final approval.

Next I had to go down to the ground floor for the assessment with the social worker. This one I felt even more at ease as I was face to face with a woman. Who knows more about the desires of being a woman than a man. Christina proceeded to discuss the same three points. But this time asking more precise questions about the surgery. There was one point she had mentioned that I had it listed as a question. She said "you do know that your new vagina is not self-lubricating?"

I replied honestly "I did not know that, but it was a question I was very curious about. She then went on to explain the next process that has to take place following the two assessments. This would be my final visit to CAMH. In a few weeks they will meet for my case meeting to decide on my approval. Next is for them to apply for government funding for the operation. Once I receive the funding approval letter. I can proceed to book my appointment with Dr. Brassard. In the mean time I could contact them to start the paperwork.

Leaving the CAMH office I felt my confidence at its peak. High on happiness I knew I was ready to take the final step to becoming a woman.

A few days later I had another beautiful moment. I was called to a problem with a machine I had in laundromat, just up the street. When I entered the laundromat I noticed only two people there. A woman and her daughter were the only ones present. I walked over to the machine unlocked it and opened the door. The little girl looked over at me and said to her Mom "she has come to fix the machine". I then overheard the mother say "yes women are clever these days they can fix things"

Hearing those words brought a smile to my face and a feeling of pride that I now belong to the female world.

After a brutal long Canadian winter, summer finally arrived. It was a bright sunny morning I had banking to do. I had decided to stay home and let Dee and Christine do my vending that day. I was preparing them to take over servicing my machines, for when I would have to recover from the operation.

I walked into the bank around the corner from me. Proceeded to the short line and looked up at the daily date sign. It was the seventeenth, my luck roulette number. "This has to be a lucky day" I thought as I moved one step closer in line. "What happiness would this day bring me?"

Arriving home after the banking I immediately went over to my desk to send an email to CAMH to ask if there was any decision, as one month had passed since my final assessment. Two hours passed when I heard my cell phone ring. It was a private number. My heart skipped a beat as I knew CAMH does not show their caller ID. It was Christine from CAMH. The words echoed through my mind. "YOU HAVE BEEN APPROVED FOR SURGERY!"

The words I so longed to hear. I thanked Christina for all she and CAMH had done for me. "You have to thank yourself, as you had done all the work," was her modest reply. I closed the phone letting out a loud "Woohoo!" Rod a friend of Dee was staying at our place at the time. He was the only other person in the condo. I ran to him telling him the awesome news. I could not hold back the tears of joy. The road had been long and winding, finally the milestone I had been longing to see. Twenty three months to the date had passed since my rebirth on 17 July 2012. Todd approached me seeing the tears of joy roll down my cheeks. "Oh girl you are emotional; let me give you a hug."

Now it was just a matter of waiting for the funding letter. At that point I could book my appointment in Montreal. Christina had informed me that they would send all the paperwork to the Dr. Brassard's clinic. Eh! My journey was finally coming closer to its destination.

I had just finished work on Monday 14 July. I entered the condo building stopping to pick up the mail. There were two brown envelops, one addressed to me and another addressed to another person but with my address. This confused me as they were both addressed from Ministry of Health. I thought it must be just another letter from Ontario Health recommending that I go for some test due to my age. I had already received one requesting I go for a pap smear as my gender is female on my health card.

I wrote RTS on the incorrect letter placed it in the RTS slot and proceeded to my condo. I was curious as to what this letter was. Sitting on my bed video camera rolling I opened the letter. I glanced at the page before turning it over to page one. When I reached the second paragraph the words jumped out at me:

"This letter is intended to confirm that, based on the documents submitted in support of your request for funding for vaginoplasty, you meet the eligibility requirements for OHIP funding and are, accordingly, approved for OHIP funding for this surgical procedure to be performed at The Centre Metropolitain de Chirurgie Plastique in Montreal, Quebec."

I shrieked with joy, knowingly that I had the expectations that I will be approved for funding. But nothing tops the actual approval in writing. I immediately scanned the letter and emailed it to the clinic. With this letter they would be able to give me the surgery date.

I realized how fortunate I am to live in a beautiful country like Canada. It was only a few years ago, 3 June 2008 that Health Insurance Act (HIA) has been amended to add sex reassignment surgery (SRS) as an insured service under the Ontario Health Insurance Plan (OHIP). This change of policy was thanks to the Ontario Liberal government.

Thursday, 17 July had arrived, would this be another lucky day? So I called up the clinic in Montreal to see how everything was proceeding. To my disappointment I was informed by the woman that the lady that handles the surgery dates was on vacation. She said she would work on my file and email me my surgery date the next day. To my disappointment no email came that Friday.

I finally heard back from the clinic about a week later after making a few phone calls to them. I even used my French speaking neighbor to call them hoping that they would be more accommodating if we spoke their native tongue. Quebec is known for their citizen's reluctance to speak English. But I did realize that the clinic deals with international patients coming to them for their gender reassignment surgery. The woman that deals with all the surgery dates was on vacation. The lady filling in for her had left me a voice message informing me that I could have my surgery 6 January 2015.

That day should have been a happy day for me. But I felt disappointed as I was determined to get my vagina for Christmas. She did inform me that I am on the cancellation list. So there is a chance of having the surgery sooner.

A few days later I received the package from them with all the surgery information and documents I would have to sign prior to surgery.

Package Document list
1. Letter of confirmation
2. Package Document list
3. Vaginoplasty
4. Medications to avoid before and after surgery
5. Preparing at home for a vaginoplasty
6. Electrolysis
7. Daily schedule in Montreal for vaginoplasty
8. Travel information
9. Specific post operative instructions
10. Specific as you heal information
11. Surgical as you heal information
12. Surgical risks for vaginoplasty
13. consent for skin graft

I was also informed to do see my Doctor to pass the following tests: CBN, BUN, glucose, urines analysis, HIV and resting EKG with interpretation. The results were valid for six months. So I managed to do all my testing early August.

12 August 2014, Tuesday

Canadian citizen test and awesome surprise: I had finally received my notice to do my citizen test, English test and documentation check. But due to a glitch in their system I had to go to their Scarborough office 150KM away, instead of the Niagara Falls office.

I had just returned home about 5pm from the two hour drive home. I sat down at my computer to catch up on any daily correspondence. The email from the clinic popped out at me:

Hi,

I have September 17th available, do you want it?

Au plaisir / With pleasure

*J**** *****

Secrétaire médicale / Medical Secretary

My immediate response was just one word "YES". I was jumping with joy at the news. Only one month away from surgery. By this time I had overcome the surreal realization I was feeling the months around my Surgery approval. I immediately grabbed my phone to text my friends. Dee was the first person I texted followed by Samantha and Christine. I heard a phone beep behind me as Dee had left her phone behind as she had stepped out to go to the supermarket.

A few minutes later Dee returned home. I was still on the phone with Samantha. I quickly said to Dee "read your message" but I could not contain my excitement "I can have my surgery next month". Hugs and congratulations all round. I could hear my computer bleeping as My Facebook post received likes from all my friends around the world. I sat down at my desk which was now relocated to the main living room area. Tears of joy steaming down my face, realizing I don't have to wait too long. Five months wait was now reduced to five weeks.

The next day I called my doctor's office to see if my test results were in. My results were in, so I instructed them to fax them over to the clinic. Once the nurse has checked that all were ok, she would fax them over. Next I had to do the travel plans for my trip to Montreal and back.

We decided on going up to Montreal by train with business class. This is a once in a life time trip. So I decided whether I cash in emergency savings or take a loan the trip up and down will be done in style. That week I sold some unused equipment and hunting gear to help cover the trip. Three of my stitches Dee, Tammy and Samantha would accompany me on this ever so important journey.

"Stitches" was a word I started to use instead of Bitch. Dee hated that word so stitch was the acceptable and preferred word to use. The word stitch also has the connotation of being attached or connected together. These were my closest girlfriends within my inner circle. These were the female friends that meant so much to me and my transition.

Now with the trip and hotel for my stitches booked, the countdown began. I had passed the stage of nervousness or worry. I was excited that finally I would have a vagina in less than four weeks' time.

For months I had planned on doing a makeover of my room. I wanted my feminine girl's room that I never had. I had two of my close female friends that had wanted to do it for me. This had created a bit of a dilemma for me. Each one of them had their own interpretation of my vision. If I had chosen one over the other I would alienate the other. So when both women were away and with the help of my male bestie Duane. I finally had my own room done to my vision. Beautiful gifts from all my girlfriends helped with the décor. From bathroom mats, a staff, candle set, fairy and Marilyn Monroe side pictures.

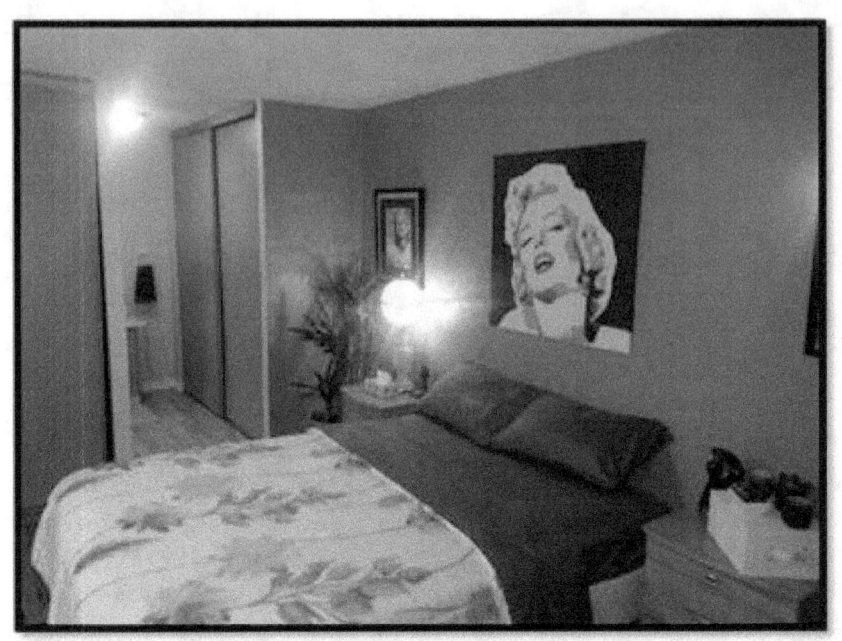

Figure 17 my beautiful feminine room

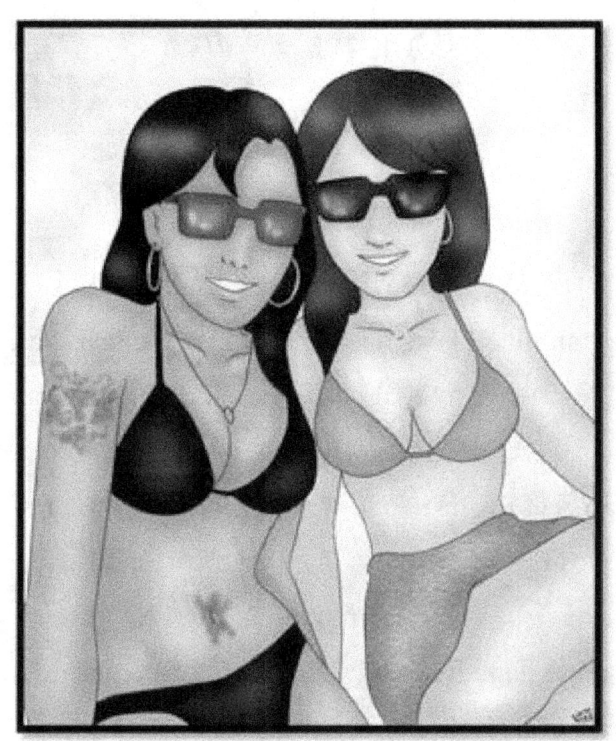

Figure 18 On the Beach Angel & Lisa

Chapter Twelve

Surgery

27 August 2014, Wednesday: With just three weeks to my surgery I had to stop taking all hormones and natural medications. So I warned my girlfriends to be prepared, if stopping the hormones might have an adverse effect on me. So I called up Vee my Mentor if she had any affect the last three weeks without hormones. I had also posed this question to the clinic that had this response
"You would have bad moods probably"
Vee on the other hand had said she felt no difference. My understanding of it, Is that it probably would have to take a while before the hormones start to wear off.

September 2014 Tuesday: A few days earlier I had received a text from my son Bret that he wanted to see me. I was immediately excited, I would see my son again. I had constantly sent him texts, without receiving any reply. It was just two weeks ago I had texted him informing him that I was to have surgery the following month. His response was like a dagger piercing my heart. I would lose him as a son forever if I proceeded with the operation. After a heart wrenching pause he followed up with the reply "do whatever makes you happy."

Even though I knew he just needed me to sign for his college funding. This was an opportunity for me to see my son again. An important opportunity for me to tell him how I truly felt. I had dropped off Dee at her niece's place. She left me with a valuable piece of advice.

"Lisa don't hold back emotions, tell him how you feel."

I parked the car at the convenience store he told me to meet him at 6pm. I had it on to me arriving there at 5:49pm. Driving over I did say a prayer, asking God to help bring my son back to me.

I looked in the side view mirror, seeing his tall slim body approaching. He was well dressed, as he entered the passenger's side. We greeted each other cordially, as he handed me over the papers to sign. I handed him a few groceries and treats I had prepared in a plastic bag for him. Without hesitation I poured my heart out to him not holding back my emotions.

He sat calmly listening to me, as I ended off asking him to try accepting me totally for who I am. We are family and I will always love him. His response comforting and understanding to me. He would try but with promises. This small but yet giant step meant so much to me. I left crying all the way back to pick up Dee. This was yet another beautiful day.

11 September 2014, Tuesday: This marked the last day I could drink alcohol before my surgery. I was informed that I must stop one week before. So this called for a case of Blue Lights, cool company and ice cold beers. Sitting on my patio with Dee we made this a special night.

14 September 2014, Sunday: Finally my crazy week came to an end. I had to prepare my business for my absence. With my bestie Christine taking the reins while I was away. After a busy last day I finally sat down at my computer to catch up on my emails. To my surprise I saw one from my brother. His words brought tears of joy and emotion.

Dear Lisa,

I believe that you are having your operation this week and want to wish you the best of luck and the operation is successful. I wish you a speedy recovery after the operation, which you will be happy and able to live the life that you want to.

Love

15 September 16, 2014, Monday: My Samsung phone alarm woke me. The day finally arrived. My bag was packed the night before. My black skirt, blue top, black panties, bra & stockings neatly piled up on the dresser. After freshening up, dressing and make up, I had to put an important call through to my parents.

I sensed from their voices over the Skype to landline, that they were upbeat about my final stage. This was comforting to me knowing my family was behind me on this important part of my journey. I hoped and wished I could have got the final blessing from my son. The night before I had sent him the text "Hi Bret remember I will always love you" hoping for some reply that never came. Nothing was going to deter me I was focused on my final stage.

Dee and Tammy accompanied me on the trip. A chilly 7am Dee and I boarded the Go Bus for Burlington, where we met up with Tammy for the Go Train to Toronto. From Toronto we were booked in business class. This was a once in a lifetime trip, so I spared no expense. Arriving at Toronto Union station we relaxed in the business class lounge before boarding the train on platform 17, my lucky number.

Along the route I was posting comments photos. I received many likes, comments and well wishes on my Facebook posts.

We had dinner at Jack Astor my treat. Pulled pork poutine was my choice. I had wanted to experience Montreal cuisine, wanting to try the Montreal smoked beef. But this was not on the menu. After dinner we were dropped off at a bar near the hotel, which happened to have a strip bar upstairs called Les Deesses. The beautiful French Canadian dancer was a delight to see. My focus was on her vagina. Admiring it knowing that in just two days I would have mine.

16 September 2014, Tuesday: I checked into the clinic at the recovery center. It was located in a beautiful part of Montreal along the Prairies River. The friendly French nurse showed me to my room on the upper level, and then took me down stairs to do the administration. 4pm I was scheduled for my first enema. So I took this wait time to site under the gazebo with Dee and Tammy. There I saw two women that had had their surgery. I took this opportunity to introduce myself to one of them, who gave me a heads up on what to expect. One woman came all the way from New Zealand to have the operation. This made me happy knowing that my surgeon was that good. Knowing well that transgender people would travel so far just to have their operation with Dr Brassard.

At 7am I was transferred over to the hospital section with another transgender woman named Gigi. There I had to go through administration once again followed by an inspection to see if I had shaved the area well enough.

The nurse had eleven years' experience. After inspecting my genitals she remarked that I would not need a skin graft as I had adequate skin. This was a major relief for me as it was my only concern I had had. Would I have enough skin for vaginal depth and vaginal lips. Once again I had to have an enema, followed by a shower using a special soap to wash from neck to knees.

17 September 2014, Wednesday: I woke up early having a good night's sleep. At 6:30am the nurse came by to instruct me to have another shower with the special soap. As of midnight I was not allowed to eat or drink, not even water. The two Surgeons passed by to check on me. I took this opportunity to ask if I am able to have my testicles placed in a jar for a souvenir. Just last night Christine had requested I give her one ball. I jokingly told her I would have it bronzed so that she could wear it on a necklace.

Unfortunately I was told that I cannot keep my balls. A while later a nurse came to see me asking if I would allow my testicles to be used for research. Well I was not able to take them as a souvenir. I decided to allow them to do so. I was paid $20 a ball.

My operation was scheduled last out of the three patients. So I had to play the waiting game. GG my awesome cool roommate went in before me. Dee and Tammy had arrived minutes before when the female nurse came for me about 11:30am. I was ready, no fear, no nervousness, I was ready.

We proceeded past the administration to the large elevator, big enough for a bed to be wheeled in. We went up one level to a small waiting room. There I had to sign another document confirming that I was to have male to female gender reassignment surgery. The nurse asked if I had seen the surgeon this morning, which I had replied "no". Soon after Dr. Brassard appeared and asked me if I was ready. To which I responded "I've been waiting for this moment all my life. I am so ready"

Minutes later we proceeded into the operating room. I was seated on the edge of the bed. Where I was made to bend my back in a hunched position and given the epidural in my spine. Followed by an injection in my IV. That was the last I could remember. The next thing I remember waking up in a big room all alone. Then I noticed two medical personnel working a few paces away. One of them came over to check on me. I might have asked how the operation went; all was a bit of a haze, which she might have responded by saying all went well and that it was over.

The two personnel wheeled my operating bed into the elevator and down to my room. We passed the administration area. I noticed Dee and Tammy, who had waited all the time at the hospital during my surgery. By this time I was aware of all my senses, even though I had read in the information that you probably won't remember much on this day.

I was not in so much pain at this time but felt the burning desire to urinate. The nurse explained to me that this is caused by the catheter, swelling and stent that were placed in my new vaginal cavity. At this point there was no euphoric moment "I have a Vagina!" Just the numbing sensation between my legs and the last groin dressing with ice packs to help combat the swelling. The stint was a condom filled with cotton wool to create a dildo vaginal cavity shape. A plastic cup mold was sewn on the front to create the external vagina shape.

I was administered two Demerol injections for pain. A few hours later Dr Brassard passed by to check on me. He informed me that the surgery was successful. That night I did not get much sleep. The constant sensation that I wanted to pee was not alleviated by the pain medication. With this unpleasant feeling I had the sensation that I still had a penis.

18 September 2014, Thursday: Day 2 post-surgery is probably the worst day I had. The constant sensation of wanting to pee was almost unbearable. The thought of having to wait four days before the stent or catheter would be removed was pure torture. The only way I was able to deal with it was to distract my mind from it or to play mind games but imagining I was peeing. This actually did make me pee at times as Dee and Tammy noticed the flow of urine to the bag. The other thought was that I was told that every day that passes brings more relief.

I had an IV connected, leg massagers to help with blood flow; the catheter; a drainage bottle connected through a needle to my inner vagina to collect the blood. The day started with a light breakfast of toast with peanut butter. For lunch I was served pasta with feta cheese and mushrooms. I did not enjoy this meal much as I am not a big lover of Italian food with the exception of alfredo dishes or pizza. Dinner was much better as I had a mushroom and meatballs. My bestie Samantha had surprised me by driving all the way from Niagara Falls just to visit me for a few hours. Holding one of the meatballs in my fork I jokingly said to her. "Look I'm having my balls for breakfast"

The staff at the hospital was totally awesome taking care of us. You could see that they all worked there as they were passionate about their job. As another transgender woman had commented, "they work from their hearts." This day I had switched to oral pain killers every four hours. This was the first night I was able to have a few solid hours sleep.

19 September 2014, Friday: What a major difference I felt. The leg massagers were the first to be removed, followed by the IV and the drainage bottle. Before I was transferred to the recovery center, scheduled for 10am. The catheter bag was removed and a valve for urinating fitted. A transgender male nurse transferred me over with a wheel chair.

This would become my home for the next seven days. It was quite the family atmosphere with other transgender patients there. We were all able to support each other. I shared a room with another woman that had her operation two days before me. So I was able to prepare myself for what I would be going through in the days to come.

20 September 2014, Saturday: Tammy and Samantha had left, so Dee had spent the day with me. I was told to take it easy over the weekend. In preparation for my dressing to be removed on Sunday and the stent removed on Monday. It was such a pleasure to have a fried egg for breakfast. Finally I was able to have a real breakfast again. At the recovery center each patient had to be more independent taking care of their dressing changes and ice pack on the groin area every hour. GG had it rough with throwing up constantly. So I had to be there to support her, at one time lying in bed with her hugging her, giving her human support.

21 September 23, 2014, Sunday: After breakfast I was relaxing in my room when the beautiful head nurse came for me. Many of the other women had commented on how beautiful she was. Just above petite size dark hair. Airing out my vagina and icing the area above my clitoris

The days, weeks and months that followed proved to be the toughest time of my life; both physically and mentally. Reflecting back at that time I realized how much I was physically and emotionally drained from the healing. I had presumed I would be healed enough after 6 weeks to return to work. But that would not be the case. My one young roommate in the recovery house said to me "If I had known what we had to go through after surgery. I would never had done it." I am sure she now appreciates that the pain and suffering she went through was totally worth it. Dilating would prove to be one of the toughest procedures that would follow. Dilating was very important to ensure that the vagina cavity does not close up.
Starting from four times a day (1-2 months). Dropping to three a day (3rd month). Twice a day (month 4-5); and eventually once a day after six months.

For the months that followed my surgery I was not able to focus on my business or continue writing this book. The only writing I did was the posts on Facebook. Here are some of the posts from myself and friends (just main posts, no comments):

Lisa Alexandra

September 17, 2014 •

Out of surgery pain but alive

Lisa Alexandra

September 17, 2014 •

I have a vagina woohoo

Like • Comment • Share

Avaya

September 17, 2014 •

I would like to congratulate my dear friend Lisa Alexandra on her new vagina today!!!!

So happy for you Lisa!!!! Can't wait to see what it looks like one day when it's all healed!!!!!

You deserved this! Was a long time coming and couldn't be happier for you!!

Love you! ! Xoxo

Lisa Alexandra

September 17, 2014 •

Just had my dressing changed. But could not see my vagina yet. They have a plastic mold sewn on to form the shape. I also have a stent inside my vagina. No pain but feel like I want to pee all the time caused by stent pushing against my bladder and the catheter

Christine

September 17, 2014 •

A big congrats to my friend on a successful surgery to a wonderful beautiful new vagina. Its all over now babe. So proud of you. Missing you like crazy but someone has to hold down the fort. Can't wait until you are home and safe and well on the way to healing. You deserve everything wonderful that has come your way. I dedicate this next post and song about vaginas to you my dear lisa. Xoxo
— with Lisa Alexandra.

Avaya Lisa Alexandra

September 17, 2014 •

Damien idea but I created it lol

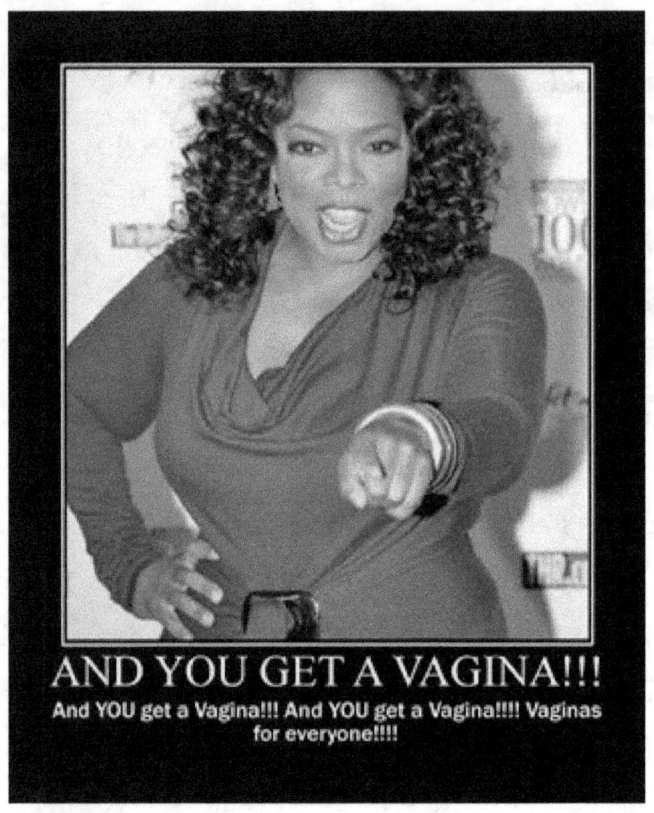

AND YOU GET A VAGINA!!!
And YOU get a Vagina!!! And YOU get a Vagina!!!! Vaginas for everyone!!!!

Lisa Alexandra

September 18, 2014 •

Awake but did not sleep till after 2pm. Had my first period lol

Lisa Alexandra

September 18, 2014 •

Just saw my surgeon. Happy to hear my surgery was a success.

Lisa Alexandra

September 18, 2014 •

Just had my first walk. Success but cannot feel the stent in my vagina opening

Lisa Alexandra

September 18, 2014 •

Ice packs on my vagina

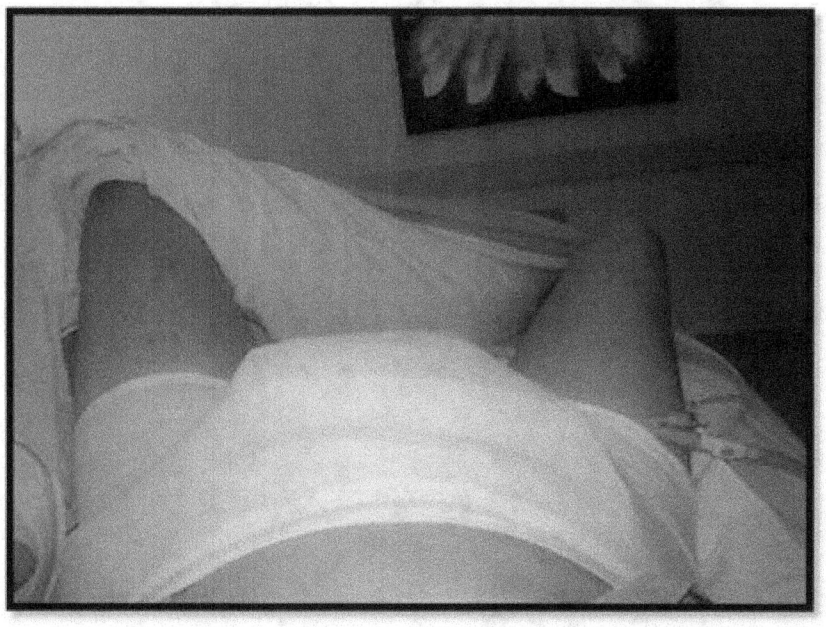

Lisa Alexandra

September 18, 2014 •

Second walk done this time 2 laps

Lisa Alexandra

September 19, 2014 •

First night since the op I was able to sleep well. Moving over to the recovery Centre today. Drainage come out today.

Lisa Alexandra

September 20, 2014 •

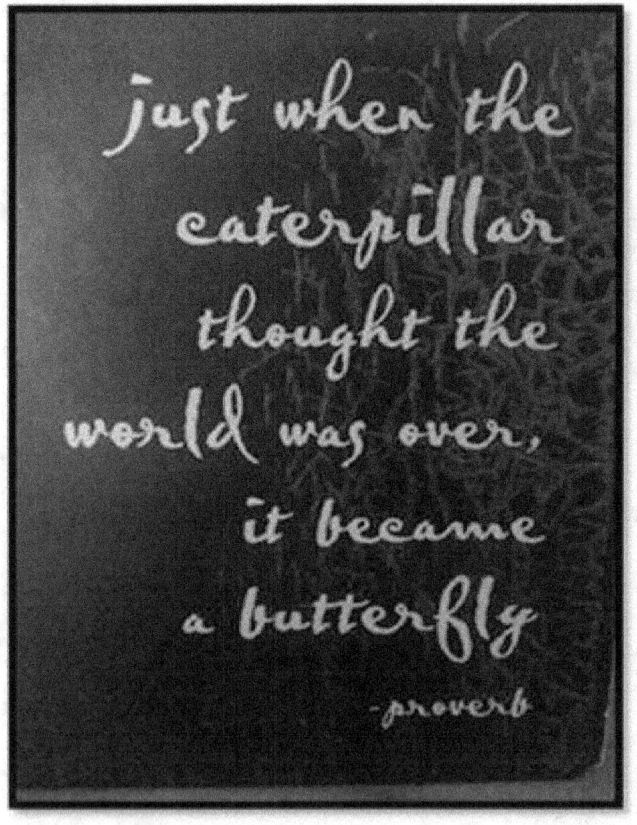

just when the
caterpillar
thought the
world was over,
it became
a butterfly

-proverb

Lisa Alexandra

September 21, 2014 •

In pain but hanging in there today I get to meet my new best friend.
Any suggestions on a cool name for my vagina?

Lisa Alexandra

September 21, 2014 •

OMG I finally got to see my vagina. Truly a beautiful moment. Even
saw the clitoris area. They say the clitoris will still blossom like a
flower. The stent is still in, so part of that is still stitched closed. But
most importantly. HAVE A VAGINA.
Crying tears of joy, the moment has finally arrived.
Dreams do come true!

Lisa Alexandra

September 21, 2014 •

Not feeling too well tonight. They say it could be because I have
been off hormones for over 3 weeks. Could be just a hot flash.
Temperature ok but pulse not.

Lisa Alexandra

September 22, 2014 •

Crazy moment, I woke up in the middle of the night with itchy balls.
I reached down only to realize nothing is there lol.

Lisa Alexandra

September 22, 2014 •

This morning Once again I awoke to the pain and realized, I just have to suck it up smile and take on the day. Today they remove the stent, so this will be a major relief.

Lisa Alexandra

September 22, 2014 •

I just had the stent removed, actually felt good; I have feelings inside my vagina.

Lisa Alexandra

September 22, 2014 •

I had my first dilation. No pain. I am surprised how deep it is. The nurse taught me about my new anatomy. This time I was really happy my vagina is looking so much more natural. I am really so impressed.

Lisa Alexandra

September 23, 2014 •

Cather removed just trying to have my first pee as a full woman.

Lisa Alexandra

September 23, 2014 •

Oohhh, so good to finally pee like a real woman. I've to get used to the

Lisa Alexandra

September 23, 2014 •

My first walk in the park with Dee
— with Dee.

Lisa Alexandra

September 24, 2014 •

Looking at the reflection in the mirror I have to say the two surgeons did an amazing work.
I have a beautiful vagina.

Lisa Alexandra

September 24, 2014 •

I had my final vagina inspection. All is good. Homewood bound tomorrow, really looking forward to seeing everyone again.

Lisa Alexandra

September 24, 2014 •

This is where all healing was done

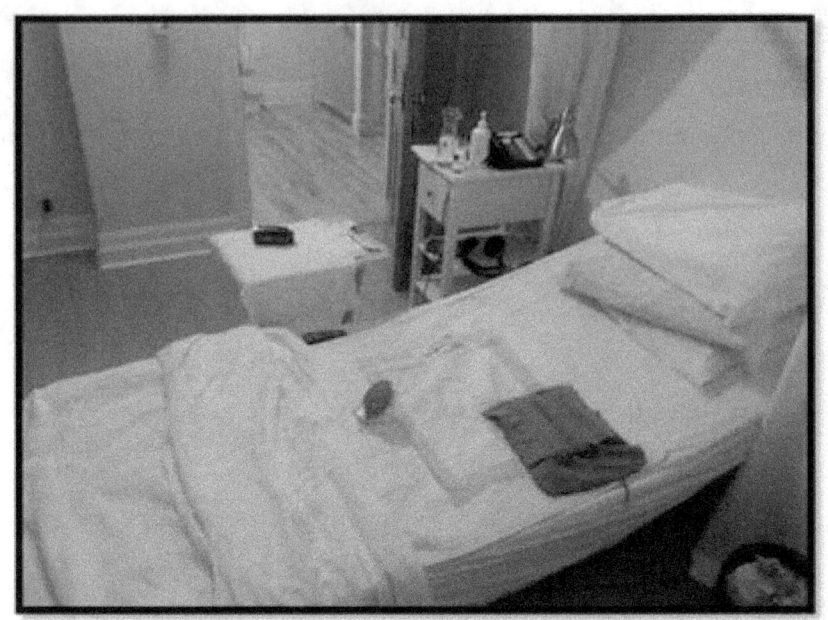

Lisa Alexandra

September 25, 2014

Homewood bound was emotional farewell to my roommate GG
together we supported each other. But most important my dream
came true I am a woman.

— with Dee.

Lisa Alexandra

September 25, 2014 •

On board for the flight to Toronto

— with Dee.

Lisa Alexandra

September 25, 2014 •

Arrived home

Lisa Alexandra

September 26, 2014 •

Day one back home. Happy I can go back on hormones. Now that the testicles are finally gone it will be interesting to see the additional effects on the estrogen.

Lisa Alexandra

September 26, 2014 •

Thank you Helen for the beautiful flowers. You made my day a beautiful one

Lisa Alexandra

September 26, 2014 •

Have to say a certain herb is helping me get through the pain and healing

Lisa Alexandra.

September 26, 2014 •

17 my lucky number

17th started my transition.

17th received my surgery approval.

Platform **17** boarded train to Montreal.

The Montreal clinic had **17** beds

17th had my surgery.

Limo driver picks me up at Toronto airport at spot **17.**

Lisa Alexandra

September 27, 2014 •

Stopped with the oxicitin yesterday. Trying to ride out the pain with just Tylenol. Tough day but I will get through it

Lisa Alexandra

September 29, 2014 •

One of the challenges since the operation. Is to retrain my brain to pee. Oh so different.

Lisa Alexandra

September 30, 2014 •

Preparing for the daily 4 dilations. Still waiting for pain to give way to pleasure.

Lisa Alexandra

September 30, 2014 •

My daily pills

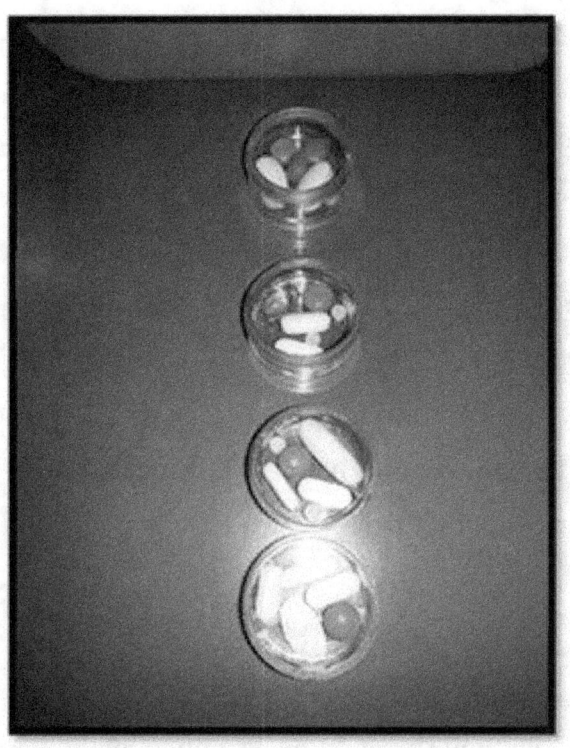

Lisa Alexandra

October 5, 2014

In becoming a woman I am experiencing pains similar to what a woman goes through at child birth and after. Not to mention my one and only period I am having. I have so much more respect and admiration for women. Lucky for me it is only once. Some of you women go thru this multiple times. As a once male I pay tribute to all women. Gentlemen admire and respect your woman as they experience much more pain than you.

Lisa Alexandra

October 10, 2014 •

Healing days are like a yoyo. One day you up next day you down. Today is an up day.

Lisa Alexandra

October 16, 2014

The butterfly is the symbol for transgender. At the moment I feel like I am still in the cocoon. But once fully healed I will emerge from this cocoon and fly free.

Lisa Alexandra

October 18, 2014

Reflecting back at my first month since my operation. Through all the pain and discomfort I have to say, I am truly happy I now have a vagina

Lisa Alexandra

October 19, 2014 •

Tomorrow I start the dreaded no. 4

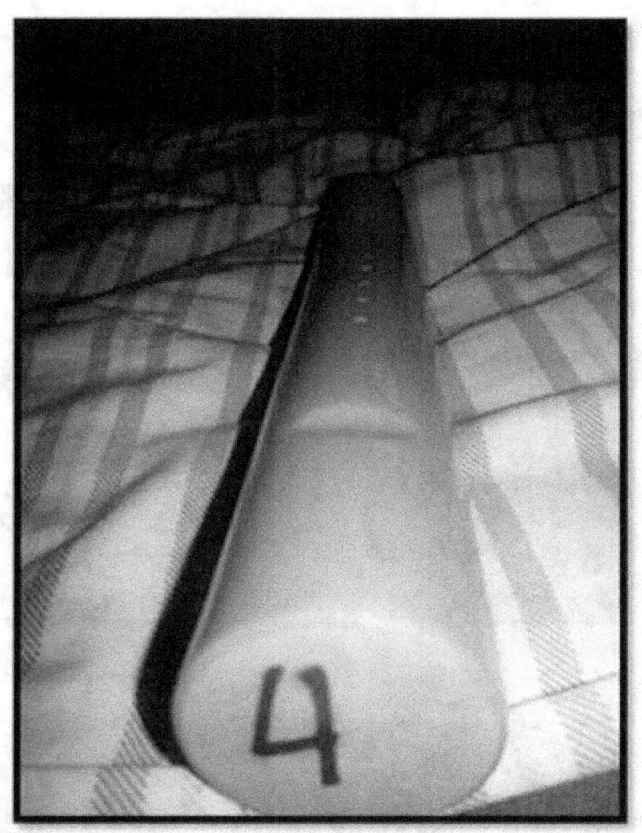

Lisa Alexandra

October 20, 2014

Omg survived the no. 4. Felt like I was violated by a donkey lol

Lisa Alexandra

October 24, 2014 •

Ready for night time dilation. Relaxing music, scents, low lights, glass of wine and plenty of lube.

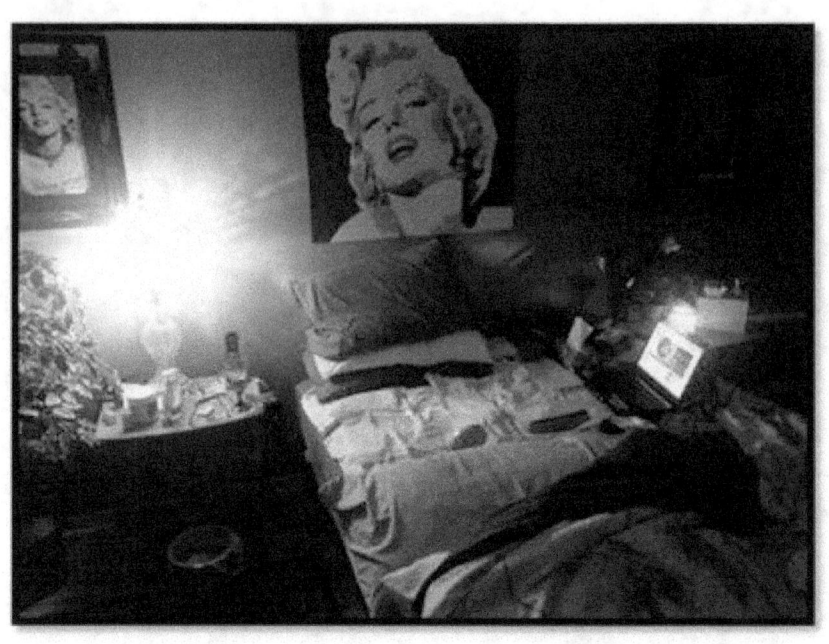

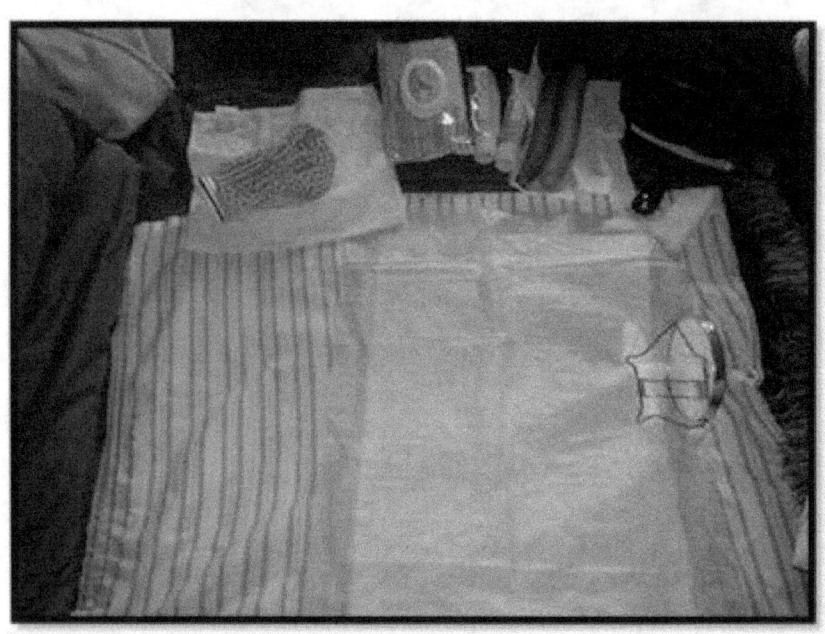

Lisa Alexandra

October 28, 2014 •

I found an interesting way to help ease my pain and progress with my healing. Watch more comedies on TV and laugh my pain away.

Lisa Alexandra

October 29, 2014

One of the questions I had at the start of my transition over 2 years ago was:

Can the hormones transform this male body to a female form?

Well I am happy to say since the removal of my last male producing hormones organ, my testicles. With full blast of estrogen. I can actually see the hour glass forming.

Oh so HAPPY!

Lisa Alexandra

October 30, 2014 •

Finally got to see the transgender doctor today for my full examination on my cookie. She said it is looking great. I feel so relieved with all the complications I have had. Besides the pain spurts I am finally feeling emotionally better.

Lisa Alexandra

October 31, 2014 •

Finally the man in the boat is starting to appear. They did say it will blossom like a flower. After two months they recommend I should start exploring it with my fingers. Just 2 weeks to go woohoo!

Lisa Alexandra

November 4, 2014 •

Sometimes the pain and discomfort out ways the will to live. But I know I must be strong and resilient. All this pain and discomfort will soon be in the past.

Lisa Alexandra

November 5, 2014 •

What a weird feeling. I now have feelings on the left side of my vagina cavity but not the right yet. Over the weekend I had some major nerve endings re-attaching. Which ads to new pains, but a good sign of healing.

Lisa Alexandra

November 9, 2014 •

Woohoo down 10 lbs post-surgery

Lisa Alexandra

November 10, 2014 •

Woohoo I finally see it for real. The clitoris is finally blooming. Nervous to touch it.

Lisa Alexandra

November 11, 2014 •

Finally noticing the swelling slowly going down.

Lisa Alexandra

November 12, 2014 •

Thank you to my stitch, bestie and fairy Christine for bringing me your shining light this morning in my darkest hour. Love you hun. I know I must be resilient as this pain, blood and discomfort will soon me in my past.

Lisa Alexandra

November 13, 2014 •

Amazing the power of friendship. Thanks to Christine Duane Samantha for making my day, yesterday and lifting my spirit. I feel so good today.

Lisa Alexandra

November 14, 2014 •

Woohoo I'm young again

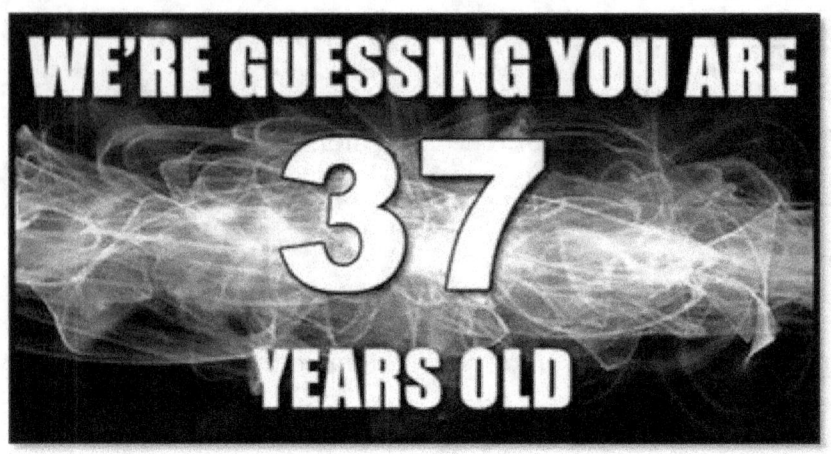

We're guessing you to be 37 years old!

Let's see if we can guess your age based on just 6 questions.

Lisa Alexandra

November 16, 2014 •

I realize why my cookie is taking strain. In the last 2 months it has been penetrated 510 times.

Lisa Alexandra

November 17, 2014 •

Today my vagina is 2 months old. One more month to go then hopefully I can return to a normal schedule.

Lisa Alexandra

December 5, 2014 •

I need batteries that have endurance. Oh soooo close!

Lisa Alexandra

December 5, 2014 •

The verdict is not in yet. So ladies I need your input and advice. Did I experience one of the three types of female orgasms?

The best way to describe it is that my body felt hypnotically paralyzed and the pleasure was endless for a few minutes. Not the release feeling that a male would experience. So my question is did I reach the top of the hill but did not get over the hill?

Lisa Alexandra

December 9, 2014 •

I'm so happy for my vagina sister Gigi, she called me joyously this morning. She finally had her big O. So happy for her, this makes all the pain and suffering so worth it.

Lisa Alexandra

December 12, 2014 •

I finally felt comfortable to shave my snatch since the operation. I think a small runway is so sexy.

Lisa Alexandra

December 13, 2014

Even though I still have some pain and discomfort. I do feel this is the turning point of my healing process. Ever so slowly normality is returning and I am starting to appreciate visually and physically my neo vagina more and more.

Lisa Alexandra

December 15, 2014 •

9 days to Christmas, still holding out hope to spend Christmas with my son. If my passport was sorted out I would have been on a plane to Africa to spend time with my family for Christmas there.

Lisa Alexandra

December 16, 2014 •

Tomorrow marks 3 months since the operation. Still bleeding, going to see my new clinic on Thursday. Hopefully they can finally help stop the bleeding. The nurse practitioner is well educated in vaginas.

Lisa Alexandra

December 17, 2014 •

I want to fall in love again for the first time.

December 17, 2014 •

Finally got to put on a pair of jeans. Oh so happy no more tucking. Today marks three months since the operation. Only problem is that I still have swelling, note the camel toe, lol.

Lisa Alexandra

December 18, 2014 •

Just got back from my first post surgery blood work. Oh wow realized how difficult it is to pee in a cup as a woman. I told the woman "you should have given me a bucket not a cup" lol

Lisa Alexandra

December 24, 2014 •

Wishing everyone a Merry Christmas with your families. I'm still holding out hope for a Christmas Miracle that I will see my son for Christmas. But if it does not happen, there are more Christmas ahead to hope for.

You added 7 new photos.

December 25, 2014 •

No son but had an awesome Christmas with friends

Lisa Alexandra

December 26, 2014 •

Truly a miracle! My son just texted me he wants to see me Sunday. So miracles do happen thank you God.

Lisa Alexandra

December 28, 2014 •

Here, goes off to pick up my son

Lisa Alexandra

December 28, 2014 •

My miracle day with my son. Thank you to Dee and Johnny for being part of this. What a beautiful day. All my dreams came true in 2014. Also thanks to Jen, thank you for being there for my son and part of this miracle.

Lisa Alexandra

January 1 •

One of my 2015 goal. To connect with as many women as possible.

Lisa Alexandra

January 8 •

My vagina sister arrives tonight. She is the one we had surgery the same day.

Harry Lisa Alexandra

January 13 •

It has been a privilege to share our experience with you each week through the courage, the pain and the tears. We are all unique individuals and have no place to judge another. Through this transition know that this was your choice and only you could make that choice. If I showed any un acceptance during your journey it would only be in love to see to it that you and Kevin are happy. I won't be able to celebrate with you as I travel from South Africa to Namibia on the 17th. I am here for you and encourage others to carry on a new relationship with you in your new life. And always remember that through Jesus I can love you and He always loves you. Your friend Harry.

Lisa Alexandra

<u>January 23</u>

On Wednesday I went into Tim Horton's, they had fresh chocolate eclairs. I just had to buy one. When I was a little girl (trapped in a boy's body), every Wednesday my Mom would go to the market and return with a chocolate eclairs for me. Yesterday when I spoke to my Mom and I told her I had bought one reminding her about the Wednesday chocolate eclairs she would buy me. I Love my chocolate eclairs.

Lisa Alexandra

<u>January 27</u> •

The joys of womanhood. My first mammogram is booked for next week.

Lisa Alexandra

<u>January 29</u> •

Woohoo received my new Dutch passport with my name and gender. Now I can finally travel free as a woman.

Lisa Alexandra

February 28 •

Sisters from a different mister at Big Texas

— with Dee.

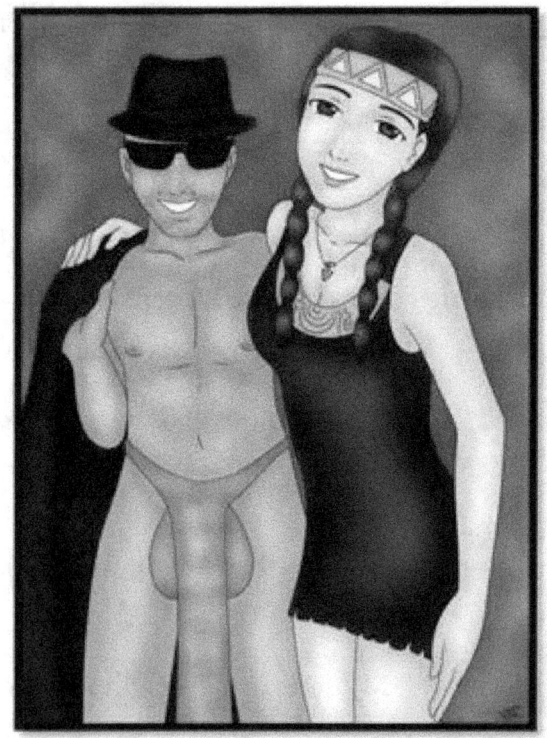

Figure 19 Halloween 2014 Mr. D & Lisa

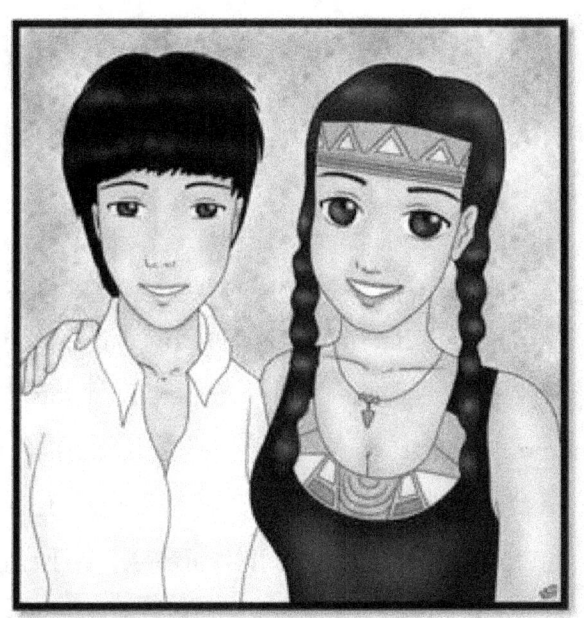

Figure 20 Halloween 2014 Miss T & Lisa

Chapter Thirteen

Finally a Woman

At the recovery center, Dee and I had met a transgender couple. The transgender woman had, had her operation over a year ago. She was there to support her transgender male partner. This was a very unique loving couple. Both were there during their GRS surgeries. He had warned Dee that the worst was yet to come. He had experienced the toughest times with his partner with her post-surgery recovery. He warned Dee that the worst was still to come with regards to me. The first three months after returning home will be the worst.

To say the least, the first four months was hell. I had totally miscalculated the healing time. I thought that I would be back to work six weeks later. GG had warned me about the addiction to Oxycodone. This was the pain medication that I had taken after surgery. Looking back at my videos I had made at the recovery center. You could see how drugged up I was. I went on the premise that we were told that most patients should stop taking pain medication when they leave the recovery center.

The days that followed the surgery I had intense pain in the clitoral area. They had kept all the nerve endings intact connected to a small portion of the head of the penis. All the nerves were folded bunched up. In time the clitoris would blossom like a flower. With all the penile nerves bunched up in one area created intense pain that not even the Oxycodone would relieve. After one week the pain would subside, but would return at unexpected times. I soon notice that when certain women were around for a visit. The pain would be intense. I soon realized that this was related to me being aroused by their presence. It was like my penis trying to become erect but was confined to a cage. I was able to cut out the Oxycodone replacing them with Tramadol. I would ease the pain with certain sensual stretches with my arms and legs. It would take months before these pains finally disappeared.

Dilation the toughest, as mentioned before this was an important procedure to ensure that the vagina cavity does not close up. We were issued with three dilators numbers 2, 3 & 4. Number 1 was not needed as the opening was large enough for the No. 2. The dilators were made of a solid hard plastic. White spots marked the various depts. The last white spot marked six-inch depth.

Dilation schedule

Month 1: 4 times per day with, #1 for 5 minutes, #2 for 15 minutes. Month 2-3: Dilate 3 times per day with #1 for 5 minutes, #2 for 10 minutes, #3 for 15 minutes.

Month 4-6: Dilate twice a day with #2 for 5 minutes, #3 for 10 minutes, #4 for 15 minutes.

Month 7-12: Dilate once a day with #3 for 5 minutes, #4 for 15 minutes.

After the first year, it drops to once a week with #4 for 15 minutes. But if you have sex with penetration, it counts as a dilation session. Dilator had to be cleaned before and after dilation with antibacterial dishwashing soap. I had settled on the green Dawn soap. You would place about a tablespoon of water soluble lubrication on the end of the dilator. KY was the preferred choice. I had tried a cheaper brand but found that the KY was the best.

The first few months were a bit painful when inserting the dilators. The trick was to try to relax your body and muscles as much as possible. I even went as far as setting up my dilation as a ritual. I would play relaxing spa music; close the curtains in the daytime or low lighting in the night; slow deep breathing. It was recommended you slowly breathe in and out ten times before you start. I would use a small electronic timer to keep time.

Douching twice a day in the earlier months was needed. After three months once a day to eventually once a week after six months. Saline water was used. This was necessary to flush the inner vaginal cavity. To clean out any dried blood or skin. As a transgender woman, it would be necessary to douche once a week for the rest of our lives. Unlike a natural born woman whose body does the cleaning naturally.

Urinating as a female would prove to be quite the challenge for me. The very first time I had peed post-surgery. Like most of my vagina sisters would say "it was like peeing through your butt." Unlike a male who pees through their penis in the front. Now all of a sudden the pee came from below. The urethra was shortened; this also made us more acceptable to unary tract infections (UTI). The anus was now closer to the urethra. We were taught after surgery that is was important to wipe from to back. Drinking plenty of water was strongly advised.

The difficult part was training the brain that the pee did not come out the front but instead below. Drink plenty of water did help in this process. Finally, after months my brain and urethra were in sync, and I was able to pee without long delays sitting on the toilet. I even had to learn the hovering technique women that they use in public bathrooms. This is when they do not want to sit down on the toilet seat. In some ways, I found it easier to pee this way.

Every person heals at a different rate, age being a major factor. The younger women would heal allot quicker. It was also important to relax and take it easy during the healing process. But it was very important to walk for at least 15 minutes four times a day. Walking would also prevent blood clotting. For the first few months, I could not sit for long periods of time. It was only after about four months that I could finally sit for longer periods than five minutes. The pressure on the neo-vagina would cause pain.

I had a complication as my stitches at the bottom of my vagina had ripped. This was possibly caused by the dilations. As the curvature of the cavity would cause the dilator to put pressure on the bottom of the vagina. This was one of the complications they had warned us about. They would not re-stitch the wound, but instead let it heal naturally. Hyper granulation had formed in the wound. This is when the flesh turns a bright red color. I had to go for silver nitrate treatments regularly to treat the area.

The nurse practitioner Christy at my local clinic in Niagara was so helpful. I would see her every two weeks for the treatment. She was well educated and had a vast knowledge of the women's anatomy. It was very interesting to learn more about my vagina from her. I was pleasantly surprised that allot of what I was going through. Natural women go through after childbirth with their vagina ripping from childbirth. I would take a tablet for pain before each treatment. The silver nitrate would burn for a few minutes. This is the same treatment used to stop nosebleeds. It would be applied by an application stick. She would use about three sticks every treatment. As the months passed, I slowly had more feelings. So these made my wound area more sensitive to the silver nitrate. It was like experiencing electric shock around my vagina as the nerves would reattach. Even though these short pains which we called "sharpies" would come and go at random times. I knew it meant the nerves were reattaching, and I was getting more feeling in and around my vagina.

This was a very difficult area to heal as the estrogen in my body would make my vagina cavity moist. Moister would cause a delay in healing. I had to air out as much as possible. This meant lying on my bed with my legs apart for long periods at a time. At first, I would do it for the recommended 15 minutes. But eventually found out that I needed to air out for longer periods like an hour.

Finally, after eight months the wound finally healed. At this time my energy level was up. The pain from my vagina was not as regular as before. I could finally start exploring my vagina. As mentioned in my Facebook post in December. I had experienced my first orgasm. It was extremely enjoyable which lasted for about fifteen seconds. It was like I had reached the top of the hill. But just could not get over the hill. I think part of this was what to expect. As a male, you would ejaculate at the time of your orgasm. I did not know what to expect. After the December experience, I took a break to heal. Exploring my clitoris back then would cause some bleeding as I was not fully healed.

At this time without the help of toys, I had discovered the right technique and positioning of my clitoris to pleasure myself. The clitoris was in some way like a smaller penis. This was achieved not by direct contact with the clitoris, but with just two fingers above it. Finally, I was able to get over the hill, and I was able to achieve full awesome female orgasms.

17 June 2015. I finally made it to the ocean on Price Edward Island. A promise I had made to myself that when fully healed I would walk along the water's edge barefoot. Feeling the waves caress my feet. Twirling around, skirt blowing in the breeze. looking out to sea. Knowing that I am finally the woman I meant to be.

Freedom day arrived on 17 September 2015. This landmark day was my first anniversary of my surgery. My vagina turned one year old! This marked freedom as dilation changed from once a day to just once a week. I was able to resort back to a normal daily schedule not having to worry about dilating every day.

My vagina had healed well except for the occasional 'sharpies' even one year later. Nerves were still reattaching. I did experience the occasional testicular pain even though they are no longer there. I contacted the clinic in Montreal to enquire why I feel this pain. The explanation I received

"Hello, Mrs. Alexandra, The cause of the pain is the retreat of the testicle. The pedicle can stay sensitive for months. You could

massage the area when you feel the pain so your body understand your new anatomy and adapt to it. The massaging of the area did bring relief to the pain."

I did appear to be calmer since the surgery. I did lack the fiery drive I had pre-surgery. Even though I was never an aggressive person, I did lack the occasional aggression I once had as a male. The lower levels of the testosterone did bring about more feminization changes. I started noticing new hair growth in areas I was losing hair before my transition. My crown which once showed balding was now filling in. My hair had grown to the longest length in my life. The gray roots were the indication of how fast my hair was growing.

Looking back at my decision I had made on 17 July 2012. I asked myself. "Lisa, do you regret your transition, now that you have gone all the way?" The answer is a firm "NO!"

But I do feel the pain I have caused my son by killing off his father. Lee is now dead and gone. I don't even think I could even try playing the male role again. We as transgender people should win an Oscar, for the cross-gender performances we had to play. All I can do is to try to be there for him whenever I can, whether it is a financial help or any advice he might want via text messaging. It is my hope that time will heal his wound and that one day he can get to know me again for the first time.

One of my biggest joys is simply slipping into a tight pair of jeans. No more tucking and concealing. I now see the smooth flatness between my legs. Losing my testicles was the most liberating physical feeling I have had. Pre-surgery I would wear long tops that would cover my genital area when wearing jeans or tights. Now I don't have to worry about having that area covered.

My only critique about my vagina is the lack of a natural woman clitoral hood. This can be corrected by a second surgery known as labiaplasty. This procedure is also done to a natural woman who wants to improve the outer appearance of their vaginas. If my finance in the future will allow this, I would seriously consider it.

I also experienced a tight feeling between the vulva slit. It felt like a tight wire pulled between my legs. One of my vagina sisters explained it this way, "It was as if they had grabbed all my junk and pulled it backward." In theory, this was in some way done. Our penile skin was inverted and stitched into the vaginal cavity. Probably giving the sensation that our penis was pulled back and up into our bodies.

It was amazing how my lucky roulette number 17 had played an important part in my journey.17 July 2012 I officially started my transgender journey.17 August 2014 I received my surgery approval. I boarded the train to Montreal at Toronto on Platform 17.17 September 2014 I had my surgery. On my return home the Limo driver picked me up at Toronto airport at spot 17. When flying to Prince Edward Island, My friend, Tammy dropped me off at Toronto Airport spot 17. Now living as a full woman, I did meet someone special to spend the rest of my life with. She so happens to be 17 years younger than me.

Looking back at my life in the Caribbean reminiscing about all the women I had sex with. I re-evaluated why I had so much sex with the six hundred plus women; searching for that tall, dark haired woman. Only to realize the woman I was searching for was me, Lisa.

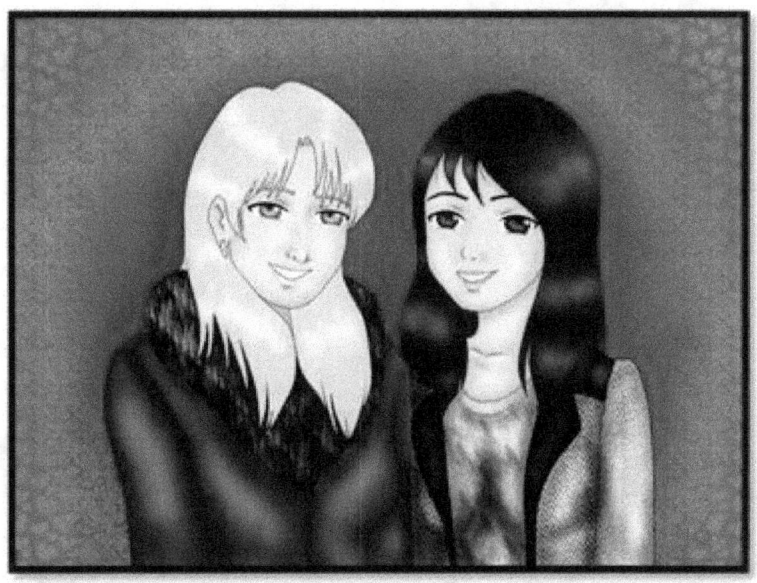

Figure 21 Lisa & her partner